W9-ATD-221

BLACKWELL'S
UNDERGROUND CLINICAL VIGNETTES

PATHOPHYSIOLOGY
VOL. II, 3E

BLACKWELL'S
UNDERGROUND CLINICAL VIGNETTES

PATHOPHYSIOLOGY
VOL. II, 3E

VIKAS BHUSHAN, MD
University of California, San Francisco, Class of 1991
Series Editor, Diagnostic Radiologist

VISHAL PALL, MBBS
Government Medical College, Chandigarh, India, Class of 1996
Series Editor, U. of Texas, Galveston, Resident in Internal Medicine &
Preventive Medicine

TAO LE, MD
University of California, San Francisco, Class of 1996

ALEXANDER GRIMM, MD
St. Louis University School of Medicine, Class of 1999

b
**Blackwell
Science**

CONTRIBUTORS

Robert Nason
University of Texas Medical Branch, Class of 2003

Tisha Wang
University of Texas Medical Branch, Class of 2002

Kristen Lem Mygdal, MD
University of Kansas School of Medicine, Resident in Radiology

Fadi Abu Shahin, MD
University of Damascus, Syria, Class of 1999

Jose M. Fierro, MD
La Salle University, Mexico City

Vipal Soni, MD
UCLA School of Medicine, Class of 1999

Hoang Nguyen, MD, MBA
Northwestern University, Class of 2001

© 2002 by Blackwell Science, Inc.

Editorial Offices:

Commerce Place, 350 Main Street, Malden,
Massachusetts 02148, USA
Osney Mead, Oxford OX2 0EL, England
25 John Street, London WC1N 2BS, England
23 Ainslie Place, Edinburgh EH3 6AJ, Scotland
54 University Street, Carlton, Victoria 3053,
Australia

Other Editorial Offices:

Blackwell Wissenschafts-Verlag GmbH,
Kurfürstendamm 57, 10707 Berlin, Germany
Blackwell Science KK, MG Kodenmacho Building,
7-10 Kodenmacho Nihombashi, Chuo-ku,
Tokyo 104, Japan
Iowa State University Press, A Blackwell Science
Company, 2121 S. State Avenue, Ames, Iowa
50014-8300, USA

Acquisitions: Laura DeYoung
Development: Amy Nuttbrock
Production: Lorna Hind and Shawn Girsberger
Manufacturing: Lisa Flanagan
Marketing Manager: Kathleen Mulcahy
Cover design by Leslie Haimes
Interior design by Shawn Girsberger
Typeset by TechBooks
Printed and bound by Capital City Press

Blackwell's Underground Clinical Vignettes:
Pathophysiology II, 3e
ISBN 0-632-04553-1

Printed in the United States of America
02 03 04 05 5 4 3 2 1

First Indian Reprint 2002

Printed and bound by Multivista Global Limited,
Chennai - 600 042.

The Blackwell Science logo is a trade mark of
Blackwell Science Ltd., registered at the United
Kingdom Trade Marks Registry

Library of Congress Cataloging-in-Publication Data
Bhushan, Vikas.
Blackwell's underground clinical vignettes.
Pathophysiology / author, Vikas Bhushan. – 3rd ed.
p. ; cm. – (Underground clinical vignettes)
Rev. ed. of: Pathophysiology / Vikas Bhushan.
2nd ed. c1999. ISBN 0-632-04551-5 (pbk.)
1. Physiology, Pathological – Case studies.
2. Physicians – Licenses – United States –
Examinations – Study guides.
[DNLM: 1. Clinical Medicine – Case Report.
2. Clinical Medicine – Problems and Exercises.
WB 18.2 B575bb 2002] I. Title: Underground clinical
vignettes. Pathophysiology. II. Pathophysiology
III. Title. IV. Series.
RB113 .B459 2002
616.07'076–dc21

2001004931

CONTENTS

ACKNOWLEDGMENTS

Throughout the production of this book, we have had the support of many friends and colleagues. Special thanks to our support team including Anu Gupta, Andrea Fellows, Anastasia Anderson, Srishti Gupta, Mona Pall, Jonathan Kirsch and Chirag Amin. For prior contributions we thank Gianni Le Nguyen, Tarun Mathur, Alex Grimm, Sonia Santos and Elizabeth Sanders.

We have enjoyed working with a world-class international publishing group at Blackwell Science, including Laura DeYoung, Amy Nuttbrock, Lisa Flanagan, Shawn Girsberger, Lorna Hind and Gordon Tibbitts. For help with securing images for the entire series we also thank Lee Martin, Kristopher Jones, Tina Panizzi and Peter Anderson at the University of Alabama, the Armed Forces Institute of Pathology, and many of our fellow Blackwell Science authors.

For submitting comments, corrections, editing, proofreading, and assistance across all of the vignette titles in all editions, we collectively thank:

Tara Adamovich, Carolyn Alexander, Kris Alden, Henry E. Aryan, Lynman Bacolor, Natalie Barteneva, Dean Bartholomew, Debashish Behera, Sumit Bhatia, Sanjay Bindra, Dave Brinton, Julianne Brown, Alexander Brownie, Tamara Callahan, David Canes, Bryan Casey, Aaron Caughey, Hebert Chen, Jonathan Cheng, Arnold Cheung, Arnold Chin, Simion Chiosea, Yoon Cho, Samuel Chung, Gretchen Conant, Vladimir Coric, Christopher Cosgrove, Ronald Cowan, Karekin R. Cunningham, A. Sean Dalley, Rama Dandamudi, Sunit Das, Ryan Armando Dave, John David, Emmanuel de la Cruz, Robert DeMello, Navneet Dhillon, Sharmila Dissanaike, David Donson, Adolf Etchegaray, Alea Eusebio, Priscilla A. Frase, David Frenz, Kristin Gaumer, Yohannes Gebreegziabher, Anil Gehi, Tony George, L.M. Gotanco, Parul Goyal, Alex Grimm, Rajeev Gupta, Ahmad Halim, Sue Hall, David Hasselbacher, Tamra Heimert, Michelle Higley, Dan Hoit, Eric Jackson, Tim Jackson, Sundar Jayaraman, Pei-Ni Jone, Aarchan Joshi, Rajni K. Jutla, Faiyaz Kapadi, Seth Karp, Aaron S. Kesselheim, Sana Khan, Andrew Pin-wei Ko, Francis Kong, Paul Konitzky, Warren S. Krackov, Benjamin H.S. Lau, Ann LaCasce, Connie Lee, Scott Lee, Guillermo Lehmann, Kevin Leung, Paul Levett, Warren Levinson, Eric Ley, Ken Lin,

Pavel Lobanov, J. Mark Maddox, Aram Mardian, Samir Mehta, Gil Melmed, Joe Messina, Robert Mosca, Michael Murphy, Vivek Nandkarni, Siva Naraynan, Carvell Nguyen, Linh Nguyen, Deanna Nobleza, Craig Nodurft, George Noumi, Darin T. Okuda, Adam L. Palance, Paul Pamphrus, Jinha Park, Sonny Patel, Ricardo Pietrobon, Riva L. Rahl, Aashita Randeria, Rachan Reddy, Beatriu Reig, Marilou Reyes, Jeremy Richmon, Tai Roe, Rick Roller, Rajiv Roy, Diego Ruiz, Anthony Russell, Sanjay Sahgal, Urmimala Sarkar, John Schilling, Isabell Schmitt, Daren Schuhmacher, Sonal Shah, Fadi Abu Shahin, Mae Sheikh-Ali, Edie Shen, Justin Smith, John Stulak, Lillian Su, Julie Sundaram, Rita Suri, Seth Sweetser, Antonio Talayero, Merita Tan, Mark Tanaka, Eric Taylor, Jess Thompson, Indi Trehan, Raymond Turner, Okafo Uchenna, Eric Uyguanco, Richa Varma, John Wages, Alan Wang, Eunice Wang, Andy Weiss, Amy Williams, Brian Yang, Hany Zaky, Ashraf Zaman and David Zipf.

For generously contributing images to the entire *Underground Clinical Vignette* Step 1 series, we collectively thank the staff at Blackwell Science in Oxford, Boston, and Berlin as well as:

- Axford, J. *Medicine.* Osney Mead: Blackwell Science Ltd, 1996. Figures 2.14, 2.15, 2.16, 2.27, 2.28, 2.31, 2.35, 2.36, 2.38, 2.43, 2.65a, 2.65b, 2.65c, 2.103b, 2.105b, 3.20b, 3.21, 8.27, 8.27b, 8.77b, 8.77c, 10.81b, 10.96a, 12.28a, 14.6, 14.16, 14.50.

- Bannister B, Begg N, Gillespie S. *Infectious Disease, 2nd Edition.* Osney Mead: Blackwell Science Ltd, 2000. Figures 2.8, 3.4, 5.28, 18.10, W5.32, W5.6.

- Berg D. *Advanced Clinical Skills and Physical Diagnosis.* Blackwell Science Ltd., 1999. Figures 7.10, 7.12, 7.13, 7.2, 7.3, 7.7, 7.8, 7.9, 8.1, 8.2, 8.4, 8.5, 9.2, 10.2, 11.3, 11.5, 12.6.

- Cuschieri A, Hennessy TPJ, Greenhalgh RM, Rowley DA, Grace PA. *Clinical Surgery.* Osney Mead: Blackwell Science Ltd, 1996. Figures 13.19, 18.22, 18.33.

- Gillespie SH, Bamford K. *Medical Microbiology and Infection at a Glance.* Osney Mead: Blackwell Science Ltd, 2000. Figures 20, 23.

- Ginsberg L. *Lecture Notes on Neurology, 7th Edition.* Osney Mead: Blackwell Science Ltd, 1999. Figures 12.3, 18.3, 18.3b.

- Elliott T, Hastings M, Desselberger U. *Lecture Notes on Medical Microbiology, 3rd Edition.* Osney Mead: Blackwell Science Ltd, 1997. Figures 2, 5, 7, 8, 9, 11, 12, 14, 15, 16, 17, 19, 20, 25, 26, 27, 29, 30, 34, 35, 52.

- Mehta AB, Hoffbrand AV. *Haematology at a Glance*. Osney Mead: Blackwell Science Ltd, 2000. Figures 22.1, 22.2, 22.3.

Please let us know if your name has been missed or misspelled and we will be happy to make the update in the next edition.

PREFACE TO THE 3RD EDITION

We were very pleased with the overwhelmingly positive student feedback for the 2nd edition of our *Underground Clinical Vignettes* series. Well over 100,000 copies of the UCV books are in print and have been used by students all over the world.

Over the last two years we have accumulated and incorporated **over a thousand "updates"** and improvements suggested by you, our readers, including:

- many additions of specific boards and wards testable content

- deletions of redundant and overlapping cases

- reordering and reorganization of all cases in both series

- a new master index by case name in each Atlas

- correction of a few factual errors

- diagnosis and treatment updates

- addition of 5–20 new cases in every book

- and the addition of clinical exam photographs within *UCV— Anatomy*

And most important of all, the third edition sets now include two brand new **COLOR ATLAS** supplements, one for each Clinical Vignette series.

- The *UCV–Basic Science Color Atlas* (*Step 1*) includes over 250 color plates, divided into gross pathology, microscopic pathology (histology), hematology, and microbiology (smears).

- The *UCV–Clinical Science Color Atlas* (*Step 2*) has over 125 color plates, including patient images, dermatology, and funduscopy.

Each atlas image is descriptively captioned and linked to its corresponding Step 1 case, Step 2 case, and/or Step 2 MiniCase.

How Atlas Links Work:

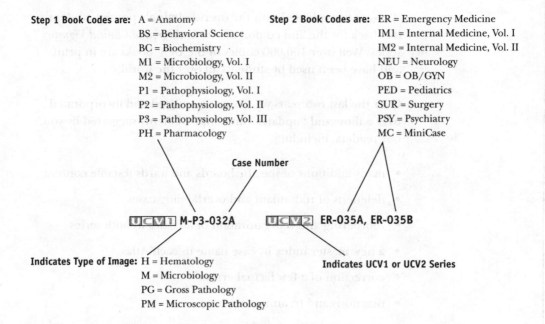

Step 1 Book Codes are:
A = Anatomy
BS = Behavioral Science
BC = Biochemistry
M1 = Microbiology, Vol. I
M2 = Microbiology, Vol. II
P1 = Pathophysiology, Vol. I
P2 = Pathophysiology, Vol. II
P3 = Pathophysiology, Vol. III
PH = Pharmacology

Step 2 Book Codes are:
ER = Emergency Medicine
IM1 = Internal Medicine, Vol. I
IM2 = Internal Medicine, Vol. II
NEU = Neurology
OB = OB/GYN
PED = Pediatrics
SUR = Surgery
PSY = Psychiatry
MC = MiniCase

Case Number

UCV1 M-P3-032A   UCV2 ER-035A, ER-035B

Indicates Type of Image:
H = Hematology
M = Microbiology
PG = Gross Pathology
PM = Microscopic Pathology

Indicates UCV1 or UCV2 Series

- If the Case number (032, 035, etc.) is not followed by a letter, then there is only one image. Otherwise A, B, C, D indicate up to 4 images.

Bold Faced Links: In order to give you access to the largest number of images possible, we have chosen to cross link the Step 1 and 2 series.

- If the link is bold-faced this indicates that the link is direct (i.e., Step 1 Case with the Basic Science Step 1 Atlas link).

- If the link is not bold-faced this indicates that the link is indirect (Step 1 case with Clinical Science Step 2 Atlas link or vice versa).

We have also implemented a few structural changes upon your request:

- Each current and future edition of our popular *First Aid for the USMLE Step 1* (Appleton & Lange/McGraw-Hill) and *First Aid for the USMLE Step 2* (Appleton & Lange/McGraw-Hill) book will be linked to the corresponding UCV case.

- We eliminated UCV → First Aid links as they frequently become out of date, as the *First Aid* books are revised yearly.

- The Color Atlas is also specially designed for quizzing—captions are descriptive and do not give away the case name directly.

We hope the updated UCV series will remain a unique and well-integrated study tool that provides compact clinical correlations to basic science information. They are designed to be easy and fun (comparatively) to read, and helpful for both licensing exams and the wards.

We invite your corrections and suggestions for the fourth edition of these books. For the first submission of each factual correction or new vignette that is selected for inclusion in the fourth edition, you will receive a personal acknowledgement in the revised book. If you submit over 20 high-quality corrections, additions or new vignettes we will also consider **inviting you to become a "Contributor" on the book of your choice**. If you are interested in becoming a potential "Contributor" or "Author" on a future UCV book, or working with our team in developing additional books, please also e-mail us your CV/resume.

We prefer that you submit corrections or suggestions via electronic mail to **UCVteam@yahoo.com**. Please include "Underground Vignettes" as the subject of your message. If you do not have access to e-mail, use the following mailing address: Blackwell Publishing, Attn: UCV Editors, 350 Main Street, Malden, MA 02148, USA.

Vikas Bhushan
Vishal Pall
Tao Le
October 2001

HOW TO USE THIS BOOK

This series was originally developed to address the increasing number of clinical vignette questions on medical examinations, including the USMLE Step 1 and Step 2. It is also designed to supplement and complement the popular *First Aid for the USMLE Step 1* (Appleton & Lange/McGraw Hill) and *First Aid for the USMLE Step 2* (Appleton & Lange/McGraw Hill).

Each UCV 1 book uses a series of approximately 100 **"supra-prototypical" cases as a way to condense testable facts and associations**. The clinical vignettes in this series are designed to incorporate as many testable facts as possible into a cohesive and memorable clinical picture. The vignettes represent composites drawn from general and specialty textbooks, reference books, thousands of USMLE style questions and the personal experience of the authors and reviewers.

Although each case tends to present all the signs, symptoms, and diagnostic findings for a particular illness, **patients generally will not present with such a "complete" picture either clinically or on a medical examination**. Cases are not meant to simulate a potential real patient or an exam vignette. All the **boldfaced "buzzwords" are for learning purposes** and are not necessarily expected to be found in any one patient with the disease.

Definitions of selected important terms are placed within the vignettes in (SMALL CAPS) in parentheses. Other parenthetical remarks often refer to the pathophysiology or mechanism of disease. The format should also help students learn to present cases succinctly during oral "bullet" presentations on clinical rotations. The cases are meant to serve as a condensed review, not as a primary reference. The information provided in this book has been prepared with a great deal of thought and careful research. This book should not, however, be considered as your sole source of information. Corrections, suggestions and submissions of new cases are encouraged and will be acknowledged and incorporated when appropriate in future editions.

ABBREVIATIONS

5-ASA	5-aminosalicylic acid
ABGs	arterial blood gases
ABVD	adriamycin/bleomycin/vincristine/dacarbazine
ACE	angiotensin-converting enzyme
ACTH	adrenocorticotropic hormone
ADH	antidiuretic hormone
AFP	alpha fetal protein
AI	aortic insufficiency
AIDS	acquired immunodeficiency syndrome
ALL	acute lymphocytic leukemia
ALT	alanine transaminase
AML	acute myelogenous leukemia
ANA	antinuclear antibody
ARDS	adult respiratory distress syndrome
ASD	atrial septal defect
ASO	anti-streptolysin O
AST	aspartate transaminase
AV	arteriovenous
BE	barium enema
BP	blood pressure
BUN	blood urea notrogen
CAD	coronary artery disease
CALLA	common acute lymphoblastic leukemia antigen
CBC	complete blood count
CHF	congestive heart failure
CK	creatine kinase
CLL	chronic lymphocytic leukemia
CML	chronic myelogenous leukemia
CMV	cytomegalovirus
CNS	central nervous system
COPD	chronic obstructive pulmonary disease
CPK	creatine phosphokinase
CSF	cerebrospinal fluid
CT	computed tomography
CVA	cerebrovascular accident
CXR	chest x-ray
DIC	disseminated intravascular coagulation
DIP	distal interphalangeal
DKA	diabetic ketoacidosis
DM	diabetes mellitus
DTRs	deep tendon reflexes
DVT	deep venous thrombosis

EBV	Epstein–Barr virus
ECG	electrocardiography
Echo	echocardiography
EF	ejection fraction
EGD	esophagogastroduodenoscopy
EMG	electromyography
ERCP	endoscopic retrograde cholangiopancreatography
ESR	erythrocyte sedimentation rate
FEV	forced expiratory volume
FNA	fine needle aspiration
FTA-ABS	fluorescent treponemal antobody absorption
FVC	forced vital capacity
GFR	glomerular filtration rate
GH	growth hormone
GI	gastrointestinal
GM-CSF	granulocyte macrophage colony stimulating factor
GU	genitourinary
HAV	hepatitis A virus
hcG	human chorionic gonadotrophin
HEENT	head, eyes, ears, nose, and throat
HIV	human immunodeficiency virus
HLA	human leukocyte antigen
HPI	history of present illness
HR	heart rate
HRIG	human rabies immune globulin
HS	hereditary spherocytosis
ID/CC	identification and chief complaint
IDDM	insulin-dependent diabetes mellitus
Ig	immunoglobulin
IGF	insulin-like growth factor
IM	imtramuscular
JVP	jugular venous pressure
KUB	kidneys/ureter/bladder
LDH	lactate dehydrogenase
LES	lower esophageal sphincter
LFTs	liver function tests
LP	lumbar puncture
LV	left ventricular
LVH	left ventricular hypertrophy
Lytes	electrolytes
MCHC	mean corpuscular hemoglobin concentration
MCV	mean corpuscular volume
MEN	multiple endocrine neoplasia

MGUS	monoclonal gammopathy of undetermined significance
MHC	major histocompatibility complex
MI	myocardial infarction
MOPP	mechlorechamine/vincristine (Oncovorin)/procarbazine/prednisone
MR	magnetic resonance (imaging)
NHL	non-Hodgkin's lymphoma
NIDDM	non-insulin-dependent diabetes mellitus
NPO	nil per os (nothing by mouth)
NSAID	nonsteroidal anti-inflammatory drug
PA	posteroanterior
PIP	proximal interphalangeal
PBS	peripheral blood smear
PE	physical exam
PFTs	pulmonary function tests
PMI	point of maximal intensity
PMN	polymorphonuclear leukocyte
PT	prothrombin time
PTCA	percutaneous transluminal angioplasty
PTH	parathyroid hormone
PTT	partial thromboplastin time
PUD	peptic ulcer disease
RBC	red blood cell
RPR	rapid plasma reagin
RR	respiratory rate
RS	Reed–Sternberg (cell)
RV	right ventricular
RVH	right ventricular hypertrophy
SBFT	small bowel follow-through
SIADH	syndrome of inappropriate secretion of ADH
SLE	systemic lupus erythematosus
STD	sexually transmitted disease
TFTs	thyroid function tests
tPA	tissue plasminogen activator
TSH	thyroid-stimulating hormone
TIBC	total iron-binding capacity
TIPS	transjugular intrahepatic portosystemic shunt
TPO	thyroid peroxidase
TSH	thyroid-stimulating hormone
TTP	thrombotic thrombocytopenic purpura
UA	urinalysis
UGI	upper GI
US	ultrasound

ID/CC An asymptomatic **60-year-old** white **male** undergoing a routine physical exam is discovered to have a **pulsating abdominal mass**.

HPI The patient has a history of **occasional abdominal pain** and **hypercholesterolemia** that has been poorly controlled by diet and medication.

PE . **Pulsating, painless upper abdominal mass** approximately 5 cm in diameter.

Imaging KUB, lateral: calcification of aneurysm wall. CT/US, abdomen: dilated aorta with irregular calcified wall; large, eccentric mural thrombus seen.

Gross Pathology Most aneurysms are located between renal arteries and iliac bifurcation; thrombus may also be present; intramural dissection may also be seen.

Micro Pathology Aneurysm wall contains all three layers (intima, media, adventitia) ("TRUE" ANEURYSM).

Treatment **Surgical replacement with graft** (if > 5 cm or symptomatic); consider endovascular stent/graft.

Discussion The risk of rupture with potentially fatal bleeding increases with size. Abdominal aortic aneurysm is usually caused by **atherosclerotic** disease and is often associated with coronary artery disease. It is also caused by trauma, infection (e.g., syphilis), **cystic medial degeneration**, and arteritis. Sequelae include rupture, embolization, infection, vascular occlusion secondary to thrombus formation, and compression of adjacent structures (e.g., ureters, vertebrae).

Atlas Link UCV1 PG-P2-001

ID/CC	A **42-year-old** white **female**, the **mother of five**, develops **acute intermittent pain in the right upper quadrant** and right scapula after eating a fatty meal.
HPI	She is of **Native American ancestry** and is 30 pounds **overweight**. She also complains of **nausea** and has **vomited** three times. She has had several prior episodes of similar pain following meals.
PE	VS: fever; tachycardia. PE: **obese**; tenderness in right upper abdominal quadrant with **inspiratory arrest on palpation** (MURPHY'S SIGN); hypoactive bowel sounds.
Labs	Hypercholesterolemia. CBC: **leukocytosis with mild neutrophilia**. Elevated direct bilirubin; **elevated alkaline phosphatase**.
Imaging	US: distended gallbladder with **wall thickening** containing **multiple echogenic shadows** (stones). Nuc, HIDA: failure to visualize gallbladder indicates cystic duct obstruction by stone.
Gross Pathology	Gallbladder inflammation ranging from wall edema to acute gangrene with necrosis, pus formation, and perforation with peritonitis. Most stones are composed of **cholesterol**; less common are **pigmented stones** made principally of unconjugated bilirubin and calcium salts.
Micro Pathology	Gallbladder mucosa contains lipid-laden foamy macrophages.
Treatment	Conservative treatment includes no oral intake, nasogastric aspiration, IV fluids, analgesics, and antibiotics; **cholecystectomy** (usually laparoscopic) is definitive treatment.
Discussion	Although calculi are involved in most cases of acute cholecystitis, **acalculous** cases arise after nonbiliary major surgeries, severe trauma or burns, and sepsis and in the postpartum state. Differential diagnosis includes appendicitis, pancreatitis, perforated peptic ulcer, pyelonephritis, myocardial infarction, and right lower lobe pneumonia. Clinical risk factors include the **four F's: fat, female, forty, and fertile**.
Atlas Link	UCV1 PG-P2-002

ID/CC A 17-year-old male student presents with **anorexia** and poorly localized **periumbilical pain followed by nausea** and two episodes of **vomiting**.

HPI Four hours after presentation, the **pain shifted to the right lower quadrant** and he developed a **low-grade fever**.

PE VS: mild tachycardia; low-grade fever. PE: **right lower quadrant tenderness with guarding and rebound**; pain in right lower quadrant when pressure applied to left lower quadrant (ROVSING'S SIGN); **pain localized to junction of outer and middle third of the line from anterior superior iliac spine to umbilicus** (MCBURNEY'S POINT); right lower quadrant pain elicited by passive hip flexion (PSOAS SIGN) and by passive internal and external rotation of hip (OBTURATOR SIGN).

Labs CBC: **elevated WBC count; predominance of neutrophils.** Normal serum amylase. UA: normal.

Imaging KUB: right psoas shadow blurred; generalized ileus with air-fluid levels; increased soft tissue density in right lower quadrant; small radiopaque **fecalith** in right lower quadrant. US: **noncompressible tubular structure** in right lower quadrant.

Gross Pathology Early lesion: hyperemic appendix with fibrinous exudate; late lesion: purulent exudate with necrosis and perforation; fecalith occasionally present.

Treatment **Appendectomy** with preoperative antibiotic coverage.

Discussion The peak incidence of appendicitis is in the second and third decades. Causes include **obstruction by fecaliths** (33%) and **lymphoid hyperplasia** (60%); it is occasionally caused by tumors (carcinoid tumor is the most common tumor of the appendix), parasites, foreign bodies, and Crohn's disease. Complications include perforation, **periappendiceal abscess**, peritonitis, and generalized or wound sepsis. Differential diagnosis should include enterocolitis, mesenteric lymphadenitis, acute salpingitis, ectopic pregnancy, pain on ovulation (MITTELSCHMERZ), and Meckel's diverticulitis.

Atlas Links UCVI PG-P2-003, PM-P2-003

ID/CC	A **67-year-old** white female complains of increasing fatigue for several months.
HPI	She has also noticed significant **weight loss** and **intermittent diarrhea**.
PE	Marked **pallor**; palpable left supraclavicular lymph node (VIRCHOW'S NODE); palpable mass in right iliac fossa; hepatomegaly.
Labs	CBC/PBS: microcytic, hypochromic **anemia. Positive stool guaiac test**; elevated serum carcinoembryonic antigen (CEA) levels.
Imaging	BE: large, irregular fungating mass in cecum. US: metastatic hepatic nodules. Colonoscopy: large fungating growth in cecum.
Gross Pathology	**Cauliflower-like, fungating, nonobstructing growth** in cecum; may be polypoid, sessile, or constricting.
Micro Pathology	Well-differentiated adenocarcinoma.
Treatment	Right hemicolectomy with temporary colostomy; adjuvant chemotherapy; follow up for recurrence by monitoring CEA levels.
Discussion	Early detection of cecal carcinoma is by screening for **occult blood in the stool**. It is the second most common cause of cancer death; its incidence increases markedly after age 50.
Atlas Link	UCVT PG-P2-004

ID/CC A 68-year-old **black male** presents with anorexia, progressive **dysphagia**, odynophagia, and **weight loss**.

HPI The patient has been drinking very **hot tea** since he was 11 years old and **smokes** one pack of cigarettes per day. His history also reveals heavy **alcohol** intake; occasional cough, vomiting, and **regurgitation**; and severe dysphagia with **solids, progressing to liquids**.

PE Emaciation; fixed, **nonpainful supraclavicular node**; pale conjunctiva.

Labs CBC/PBS: hypochromic, microcytic anemia. Hemoccult-positive stool; hypoalbuminemia.

Imaging UGI: **irregular fungating esophageal mass** in middle third of esophagus with partial obstruction. CT, chest: irregular esophageal mass with invasion of mediastinum and enlarged para-aortic lymph node.

Gross Pathology Large fungating mass protruding toward esophageal lumen.

Micro Pathology Squamous cell carcinoma on biopsy.

Treatment Laser ablation of tumor with palliative stent placement; palliative radiotherapy; surgical resection followed by chemotherapy plus radiotherapy for curable tumors; eventual gastrostomy tube placement.

Discussion The most common variant of esophageal carcinoma is **squamous cell carcinoma**, which is associated with alcohol and tobacco use and is more common in blacks. A less common variant is **adenocarcinoma**, which usually involves the distal third of the esophagus and is more common in whites with **Barrett's** (glandular metaplasia of the squamous epithelium of the distal esophagus is caused by chronic, untreated gastroesophageal reflux disease).

Atlas Links 🅄🅒🅥🅸 PG-P2-005A, PG-P2-005B

ESOPHAGEAL CARCINOMA

ID/CC	An 83-year-old white male complains of **anorexia, frequent vomiting**, and a **gnawing midepigastric pain** of several months' duration.
HPI	The pain is **not relieved by antacids or milk**. The patient has **lost significant weight** over the past few months due to diarrhea after every meal.
PE	Pale, **emaciated** male in moderate distress; left supraclavicular lymph node (VIRCHOW'S NODE) palpable.
Labs	CBC: **hypochromic, microcytic anemia**. Stool **positive for occult blood**; LFTs normal.
Imaging	UGI: large fungating lesion on greater curvature of stomach with fistulous tract running to transverse colon. EGD: same.
Gross Pathology	Polypoid, raised, fungating mass projecting into lumen; situated at distal end of stomach.
Micro Pathology	Biopsy reveals a **well-differentiated adenocarcinoma** with **signet-ring** cells.
Treatment	Surgery; radiotherapy; chemotherapy.
Discussion	Most commonly found on the **lesser curvature** in the **antrum** and **pyloric areas**, adenocarcinomas may be one of two types: **intestinal** and **diffuse**. Chronic atrophic gastritis, pernicious anemia, infection with *H. pylori*, postsurgical gastric remnants, and type A blood are all predisposing risk factors for the development of adenocarcinoma. It most commonly spreads hematogenously to the liver and may spread transperitoneally to the ovaries (KRUKENBERG TUMOR).
Atlas Link	UCV1 PG-P2-006

ID/CC	A 44-year-old male is admitted to the hospital following episodes of **vomiting blood** (HEMATEMESIS) and passing **black, tarry, foul-smelling stools** (MELENA).
HPI	He has experienced **recurrent painless hematemesis** and **melena** for several years, but repeated evaluations have been negative.
PE	Pallor.
Labs	CBC: **microcytic, hypochromic anemia**. Nasogastric aspirate has **coffee-ground** appearance.
Imaging	UGI/EGD: 5-cm mass in fundus of stomach with 2-cm ulcer on surface.
Gross Pathology	Postoperative specimen reveals a firm, circumscribed nodular **mass within the gastric wall** covered by mucosa.
Micro Pathology	Whorling interlaced bundles of spindle-shaped cells; no evidence of anaplasia.
Treatment	Surgical resection.
Discussion	Gastric leiomyoma is the **most common benign tumor of the stomach**.

ID/CC	A 40-year-old male presents with **cramping abdominal pain** and **vomiting** of 3 hours' duration.
HPI	He also complains of an **inability to pass stool or flatus** (OBSTIPATION) for the past 3 days. Two years ago, he underwent an emergency appendectomy for a ruptured appendix.
PE	Dehydration; **abdominal distention**; generalized mild tenderness over abdomen without rebound or guarding; bowel sounds heard as **high-pitched tinkles during pain paroxysms**.
Labs	CBC/PBS: leukocytosis with hemoconcentration. Serum amylase levels normal.
Imaging	XR, abdomen: "stepladder" pattern of multiple **dilated loops of small bowel** and **multiple air-fluid levels; colon and rectum gasless** (air in colon or rectum would indicate an intestinal ileus); no free air under diaphragm.
Treatment	IV fluid and electrolyte replacement; nasogastric suction/decompression; broad-spectrum antibiotics; surgery.
Discussion	The most common causes of small bowel obstruction are intestinal **adhesions secondary to prior abdominal surgery, intussusception, volvulus**, and incarcerated **hernia**; the most common causes of large bowel obstruction are **carcinoma, volvulus**, and **sigmoid diverticulitis**. Complications include **strangulation** and **necrosis** of the bowel wall leading to perforation, peritonitis, sepsis, and shock.

INTESTINAL OBSTRUCTION—ACUTE

ID/CC An **18-month-old male** is brought to the emergency room by his parents because of acute, **intermittent abdominal pain**, abdominal distention, and passage of **"red currant jelly" stools**.

HPI The child had previously been well, and his immunization schedule is complete. He **vomited** twice following admission.

PE Child crying and screaming, with knees drawn to abdomen; abdomen tender and distended; **oblong** (sausage-shaped) **mass** in abdomen (most often in right upper quadrant) that hardens with palpation; examining finger stained with **mucus and blood** on digital rectal examination.

Labs No parasites on stool exam; no pathogen on stool culture.

Imaging XR, abdomen: gas in small intestine and absence of cecal gas shadow. BE: **telescoping** of ileum into cecum.

Gross Pathology During operation, three layers are seen: entering or inner tube, returning or middle tube, and sheath or outer tube; outer tube called intussuscipiens; inner and middle together called intussusceptum.

Micro Pathology **Ischemic necrosis** with sloughing of mucosa, producing "red currant jelly" stools.

Treatment Hydrostatic (barium) or pneumatic (air) **reduction** using an enema; surgical reduction or resection if that fails or is contraindicated owing to perforation or gangrene.

Discussion Ninety-five percent of cases of intussusception are idiopathic and usually originate near the ileocecal junction. The condition is associated with adenovirus infections, which produce **hyperplasia of Peyer's patches** in the terminal ileum, which serves as a nidus for intussusception. It is also seen with **lead points** (e.g., Meckel's diverticulum, polyps, parasites, duplications, hemangiomas, and suture lines).

Atlas Link [UCV1] PG-P2-009

INTUSSUSCEPTION

ID/CC	A 51-year-old male complains of **pruritus** and **abdominal pain** that **radiates to his back** along with **significant weight loss** (15 kg) over the past 4 months.
HPI	He also states that his **urine is dark** and that his **stools are clay-colored** (ACHOLIC). He admits to a history of **smoking** (60 pack-years) and heavy alcohol use with **multiple prior bouts of pancreatitis**.
PE	**Cachectic** male; **scleral icterus** (indicates **jaundice**); **hepatomegaly; palpable gallbladder** (COURVOISIER'S SIGN); hard 8-cm mass palpable in **midepigastric** region.
Labs	**Markedly elevated direct bilirubin** (20 mg/dL); absence of urinary urobilinogen; markedly **elevated alkaline phosphatase**; mildly elevated transaminases; normal PT; **elevated carcinoembryonic antigen (CEA) and CA 19-9**.
Imaging	CT/US: **mass in head of pancreas; dilated intrahepatic bile ducts**. ERCP: abrupt cutoff of main pancreatic duct. UGI: narrowed lumen of duodenum.
Gross Pathology	Hard nodular mass with ill-defined borders invading pancreatic parenchyma and **obstructing common bile duct** around head of pancreas with local extension and liver metastases.
Micro Pathology	Pancreatic mass biopsy reveals a poorly differentiated **ductal adenocarcinoma** in clusters, secreting mucin and dense collagenous desmoplastic stroma.
Treatment	Surgical pancreaticoduodenectomy (WHIPPLE'S PROCEDURE); chemotherapy; supportive and palliative care (biliary decompression to relieve jaundice; celiac plexus block for pain).
Discussion	Chronic gallbladder disease, diabetes mellitus, hereditary pancreatitis, **chronic pancreatitis, cigarette smoking**, diets high in meat and fat, and occupational exposure to **carcinogens** are predisposing factors. Pancreatic carcinoma carries a **poor prognosis** (85% are already locally invasive or metastatic at the time of diagnosis) and is associated with a mutation in the K-ras oncogene and the p53 tumor suppressor gene. Complications include hypercoagulability (resulting in **migratory thrombophlebitis**, also known as the Trousseau sign).
Atlas Link	UCV1 PG-P2-010

ID/CC A newborn girl is brought into the genetics department for a karyotype study.

HPI She was born of a **45-year-old mother** who feels that her child is **developmentally retarded** with **characteristic "mongoloid" facial features**; her pregnancy was uneventful.

PE Generalized **hypotonia**; flattened face and low-set ears; **macroglossia**; flattened nasal bridge and **epicanthal folds**; silver-white spots on the periphery of irises (BRUSHFIELD SPOTS); single **transverse palmar crease** (SIMIAN CREASE); widely split fixed S2 (due to an atrial septal defect).

Labs Karyotype: **47,XX; trisomy 21**.

Imaging KUB: **double bubble** (dilated stomach and proximal duodenum) due to **duodenal atresia**. XR, plain: hypoplastic middle and terminal phalanges of fifth digits (ACROMICRIA).

Gross Pathology Brachycephalic head; small brain with shallow sulci; hypoplasia of frontal sinuses; endocardial cushion defect.

Treatment Surgery for congenital heart defects and duodenal atresia; training in specialized groups.

Discussion The **most common chromosomal disorder**, Down's syndrome is most frequently caused by trisomy 21 (due to nondisjunction); it is less commonly caused by mosaicism or a Robertsonian translocation. It is associated with a higher incidence with **advanced maternal age** (indication for prenatal screening); a higher incidence of cardiac defects, especially **endocardial cushion defects**; and a higher incidence of **acute lymphocytic leukemia** and **presenile dementia of Alzheimer's type**.

ID/CC	A 7-year-old boy is brought to the optometrist for **diminished visual acuity** and requests a prescription for eyeglasses.
HPI	The boy has an unusual body habitus with long arms and legs; a family history reveals similar body proportions in other family members. He is referred to his family doctor, who on careful questioning discloses that an **uncle died** of a **ruptured aortic aneurysm**.
PE	Tall; **long extremities**; arm span greater than height (DOLICHOSTENOMELIA); **long, slender fingers** (ARACHNODACTYLY); **dislocation of lenses** (ECTOPIA LENTIS); severe myopia; inguinal hernia; high-arched palate; flat feet (PES PLANUS); **aortic diastolic murmur** (aortic insufficiency); funnel chest due to pectus excavatum; scoliosis of thoracic spine.
Labs	Increased urinary hydroxyproline.
Imaging	CXR/CT/MR: marked dilatation of ascending aorta. XR, plain: thoracic and lumbar kyphoscoliosis. Echo: **mitral valve prolapse**.
Micro Pathology	**Cystic medial necrosis** of aorta may lead to **dissection, rupture, aneurysm**, or **aortic insufficiency**; elastic lung fibers tortuous and thickened; emphysema formation.
Treatment	Spine bracing; ophthalmologic correction; endocarditis prophylaxis; β-adrenergic blockers; aortic valve replacement.
Discussion	A systemic connective tissue disease characterized by an **autosomal-dominant** pattern of inheritance, Marfan's syndrome is due to a defective chromosome 15 **fibrillin gene**, a glycoprotein secreted by fibroblasts that acts as a scaffolding for the deposition of elastin.
Atlas Link	UCV2 IM2-011

ID/CC	A **5-year-old white** female is brought to her pediatrician because of fever, **marked weakness, pallor, bone pain**, and bleeding from her nose (EPISTAXIS).
HPI	She has a history of progressively increasing fatigability and **recurrent infections** over the past few months.
PE	VS: fever. PE: marked pallor; epistaxis; ecchymotic patches over skin; **sternal tenderness**; slight hepatosplenomegaly with **nontender lymphadenopathy**; no signs of meningitis; normal funduscopic exam.
Labs	CBC/PBS: normocytic, normochromic **anemia; absolute lymphocytosis with excess blasts** (> 30%) **and neutropenia; thrombocytopenia**. Common acute lymphoblastic leukemia antigen **(CALLA)** (CD10) **positive**; terminal deoxytransferase **(TDT) positive** (marker of immature T and B lymphocytes) on enzyme marker studies; negative monospot test for Epstein-Barr virus.
Imaging	CXR: no lymphadenopathy.
Gross Pathology	Neoplastic infiltration of lymph nodes, spleen, liver, and bone marrow with loss of normal architecture.
Micro Pathology	**Myelophthisic bone marrow** (distorted architecture secondary to space-occupying lesions) with lymphoblastic infiltration; lymphoblasts with inconspicuous nucleoli, condensed chromatin, and scant cytoplasm.
Treatment	Treat infection with antibiotics, **anemia** with blood transfusions, **thrombocytopenia** with platelet concentrations. Remission induction and consolidation chemotherapy. Consider bone marrow transplant.
Discussion	Acute lymphocytic leukemia (ALL) is the **most common pediatric neoplasm**; it accounts for 80% of all childhood leukemias. It carries a **good prognosis**.
Atlas Links	UCV1 H-P2-013A, H-P2-013B, H-P2-013C

ACUTE LYMPHOCYTIC LEUKEMIA (ALL)

ID/CC	A **25-year-old woman** presents with **high-grade fever, menorrhagia**, and marked weakness.
HPI	Over the past several weeks, she has also had **recurrent infections**.
PE	Marked **pallor**; multiple purpuric patches over skin; hepatosplenomegaly; **gingival hyperplasia**; sternal tenderness; normal funduscopic and neurologic exam.
Labs	CBC/PBS: normocytic, normochromic **anemia; thrombocytopenia**; leukocytosis composed mainly of **myeloblasts and promyelocytes** (nonmaturing, early blast cells); **neutropenia**. Prolonged PT and PTT.
Gross Pathology	Bone erosion due to **marrow expansion**; chloroma formation, mainly in skull; splenomegaly.
Micro Pathology	Myeloblasts with myelomonocytic differentiation replace normal marrow (MYELOPHTHISIC BONE MARROW); **basophilic cytoplasmic bodies** (AUER RODS) in myelocytes; **peroxidase-positive** stains on bone marrow and gingival biopsy.
Treatment	Chemotherapy; all-trans retinoic acid in acute promyelocytic leukemia; bone marrow transplant during first remission if HLA-matched donor available.
Discussion	Acute myelogenous leukemia (AML) is not as common in children as is ALL. An increased risk is associated with ionizing radiation, benzene exposure, Down's syndrome, and cytotoxic chemotherapeutic agents.
Atlas Links	UCVI H-P2-014A, H-P2-014B, H-P2-014C, H-P2-014D

ID/CC A 12-year-old male presents with high fever, marked **pallor**, and **epistaxis**; he has a history of **recurrent URIs** and high-grade fever that have been treated with parenteral antibiotics.

HPI He has also shown **marked weakness** over the past 3 months. He lives in the vicinity of an industrial unit that handles petroleum distillates such as **benzene**.

PE VS: fever. PE: marked pallor of skin and conjunctiva; oral and nasal mucosal **petechiae; purpuric patches** visible on skin; no significant lymphadenopathy; **no hepatosplenomegaly**.

Labs CBC/PBS: **anemia, neutropenia, and thrombocytopenia** (PANCYTOPENIA); anemia with low reticulocyte count; normal RBC morphology. Normal serum bilirubin; negative Coombs' test; normal chromosomal studies.

Gross Pathology Increased yellow marrow and decreased red marrow.

Micro Pathology Hypocellular bone marrow with empty spaces populated by fat cells, fibrous stroma, and scattered lymphocytes; marked decrease in all cell lines.

Treatment Removal of myelotoxin (in this case, benzene); bone marrow transplantation; immunosuppressive treatment with anti-thymocyte globulin; myeloid growth factors (e.g., GM-CSF) for neutropenia.

Discussion Sixty-five percent of cases are **idiopathic**. Aplastic anemia following **drug or toxin exposure** may be dose dependent (e.g., benzene, cytotoxic drugs, radiation) or idiosyncratic (e.g., chloramphenicol). Other causes include **viral infection** and Fanconi's anemia, an autosomal-recessive disorder in DNA repair.

Atlas Link UCV1 H-P2-015

ID/CC	A 66-year-old white man recently **diagnosed with chronic lymphocytic leukemia** comes into the emergency room complaining of **fatigue** and tachycardia.
HPI	He also states that his **urine** has been progressively turning **dark and red** over the course of the day.
PE	VS: tachycardia. PE: dyspnea; pallor of skin and mucous membranes; slight jaundice; **splenomegaly**.
Labs	CBC/PBS: **severe anemia; positive Coombs' test; reticulocytosis;** spherocytosis; "bite cells." UA: hemoglobinuria. Increased serum indirect bilirubin.
Gross Pathology	Congestive splenomegaly (due to **extravascular hemolysis** in the spleen).
Treatment	Prednisone; transfusions; splenectomy; immunosuppressive drugs. Discontinue any offending drug.
Discussion	Autoimmune hemolytic anemia is idiopathic in about 50% of cases; it is characterized by autoantibodies against RBC membranes (Rh), complement activation, and phagocytosis of RBCs by splenic macrophages. Three main types exist: **warm antibody** (80% to 90%; associated with leukemia, lymphoma, SLE, and viral infections); **cold reacting antibody** (10%; associated with EBV/mycoplasma infections and lymphoma); and **drug-induced** (methyldopa, quinidine, penicillin).
Atlas Link	UCV1 H-P2-016

ID/CC   A 35-year-old woman is admitted to the hospital with **left-sided weakness upon awakening**.

HPI   She has **no history** of prior headaches, seizures, hypertension, or diabetes and neither smokes nor takes drugs. Her **first three pregnancies** were **spontaneously aborted**; the fourth resulted in **unexpected fetal death**.

PE   VS: normal. PE: patient conscious; mild pallor; **left hemiplegia** with exaggerated deep tendon reflexes and extensor plantar response (POSITIVE BABINSKI'S SIGN); no neck rigidity; fundus normal; no carotid bruit; no cardiac murmurs; **reddish-blue mottling of skin in fishnet pattern** (LIVEDO RETICULARIS) on extremities; positive Homans' sign in left leg.

Labs   CBC: mild thrombocytopenia. **Prolonged PTT**; normal bleeding and clotting times; **false-positive VDRL** (titer < 1:18); FTA-ABS for syphilis negative; ELISA shows presence of **anticardiolipin antibody (ACA)**.

Imaging   CT, head (24 hours later): hypodensity (due to infarct) in right internal capsule.

Treatment   **Anticoagulant therapy** with heparin; use of **low-dose aspirin and heparin**, either alone or in combination with **prednisone**, is advocated during pregnancy in cases with a **complicated obstetric history** (e.g., spontaneous abortions or intrauterine demise).

Discussion   The presence of **lupus anticoagulant** and **ACA** defines antiphospholipid syndrome; it is further characterized by **recurrent deep venous thrombosis** in the lower extremities, thrombosis in the renal and hepatic veins, **pulmonary hypertension, cerebral artery occlusion** associated with stroke and transient ischemic attacks (TIAs), and neurologic findings that resemble multi-infarct dementia or epilepsy.

ANTIPHOSPHOLIPID ANTIBODY SYNDROME

ID/CC	A **9-year-old** girl, the daughter of **African** immigrants, presents with a large **swelling of the left side of her face and jaw** of **3 weeks' duration**.
HPI	Two weeks ago, she complained of **loosening of the** upper second left **molar**. Despite the size of the tumor, there is **no pain** associated with it.
PE	Pallor; large, firm, ill-defined **mass** encompassing entire **upper mandible**, producing mild ipsilateral exophthalmos with **deformation** on left side of face.
Labs	CBC/PBS: normocytic, normochromic anemia; mild leukopenia; positive direct Coombs' test. Karyotype: chromosomal translocation **t(8;14)** involving c-myc gene.
Imaging	CXR: no evidence of mediastinal widening (vs. Hodgkin's lymphoma).
Gross Pathology	Firm, ill-defined tumor involving upper mandible and deforming neighboring structures, but **no ulceration** or necrosis; **no satellite adenopathy**.
Micro Pathology	Giemsa-stained FNA shows cells of uniform size with nongranular basophilic nuclei and some vacuoles, 2 to 5 nucleoli, and evenly distributed chromatin surrounded by small, thin, eccentric cytoplasm that is pyroninophilic; **high mitotic index** and typical **"starry sky"** image pattern (due to diffuse distribution of macrophages among tumor cells).
Treatment	High-dose, short-term chemotherapy; alkalinize urine, force diuresis; bone marrow transplantation; intrathecal methotrexate for meningeal prophylaxis.
Discussion	Burkitt's lymphoma is a small noncleaved lymphoma **(non-Hodgkin's lymphoma)**. It is a poorly differentiated **B-cell** lymphoblastic lymphoma. The endemic (African) form is characterized by jaw tumors and is associated with **EBV** infection; the nonendemic (Western) form is characterized by abdominal and pelvic involvement. The condition was first described by Denis Burkitt in 1958 in Uganda.
Atlas Link	UCV2 Z-P2-018

ID/CC	A **65-year-old male** visits his family doctor for a routine annual checkup.
HPI	On directed history, he admits to a **weight loss** of about 12 pounds over the past 4 months, together with episodes of **epistaxis** and extreme **fatigue**.
PE	Generalized nontender **lymphadenopathy**; pallor; **enlargement of spleen and liver**.
Labs	CBC/PBS: **markedly elevated WBC count** (124,000); **90% lymphocytes**; no lymphoblasts; mild thrombocytopenia; **Coombs-positive hemolytic anemia; smudge cells** (fragile lymphocytes).
Imaging	CT/US: hepatosplenomegaly.
Gross Pathology	Lymph node enlargement almost always present; hepatosplenomegaly with tumor nodule formation.
Micro Pathology	Bone marrow biopsy reveals extensive infiltration, mainly by normal-looking lymphocytes and a few lymphoblasts with small, dark, round nuclei and scant cytoplasm; liver, spleen, lymph node involvement common; B lymphocytes fail to mature properly.
Treatment	Chemotherapy; prednisone or splenectomy for complications such as autoimmune hemolytic anemia or immune thrombocytopenia.
Discussion	Chronic lymphocytic leukemia (CLL) is a malignant neoplastic disease of **B lymphocytes** that express the surface marker CD5 (usually in T lymphocytes); it is characterized by **slow progression** of anemia, hemolytic anemia, recurrent infections, lymph node enlargement, and bleeding episodes.
Atlas Link	UCV1 H-P2-019

HEMATOLOGY/ONCOLOGY

ID/CC	A 40-year-old white male visits a doctor for a life insurance physical examination.
HPI	The patient has no major complaints except for occasional **fatigue** (due to hypermetabolic state) and **increasing abdominal girth** (due to enlarged spleen).
PE	Pallor of skin and mucous membranes; **markedly enlarged spleen; pain on palpation over sternum** (due to marrow overexpansion); no lymphadenopathy; no other abnormalities found.
Labs	CBC/PBS: **markedly elevated WBC count** (130,000); immature granulocytes mixed with normal-appearing ones; **basophilia**; eosinophilia; early thrombocytosis; late thrombocytopenia. **Low leukocyte alkaline phosphatase**; elevated serum vitamin B$_{12}$ level. Karyotype: chromosomal translocation **t(9;22)/bcr-abl gene** (PHILADELPHIA CHROMOSOME).
Imaging	US, abdomen: splenomegaly.
Gross Pathology	Skull chloromas (malignant, green-colored tumor arising from myeloid tissue); enlarged and congested spleen with areas of thrombosis and microinfarcts; hepatomegaly (due to proliferation and infiltration by granulocyte precursors and mature granulocytes).
Micro Pathology	Hepatic sinusoidal leukemic infiltrates; congestive splenomegaly with myeloid metaplasia; Philadelphia chromosome in all myeloid progeny.
Treatment	Hydroxyurea; α-interferon; leukapheresis; bone marrow transplantation (the only potentially curative treatment). Treatment ineffective after development of blast crisis.
Discussion	In chronic myelogenous leukemia (CML), death usually results from accelerated transformation into acute leukemia (BLAST CRISIS) within 2 to 5 years.
Atlas Links	[UCVI] H-P2-020A, H-P2-020B

ID/CC	A 55-year-old male presents with **swelling, pain**, and **redness** of the right **leg**.
HPI	He is retired and leads a **sedentary lifestyle**. He admits to a 70-pack-year smoking history and occasional alcohol intake.
PE	VS: fever (38.4°C); tachycardia (HR 106); mild hypertension (BP 142/92); normal RR. PE: right **lower extremity swollen; pain** elicited on **calf palpation** and on **dorsiflexion** of right foot (HOMANS' SIGN).
Labs	Blood **D-dimer elevated**.
Imaging	US, Doppler: **thrombi occluding right common femoral and popliteal veins**. Venography: **gold standard** for diagnosis, but rarely indicated.
Treatment	**Anticoagulation** with IV heparin, followed by long-term anticoagulation with oral warfarin or subcutaneous low-molecular-weight heparin.
Discussion	Virchow's triad **(venous stasis, vessel wall injury, and hypercoagulable state)** contributes to the formation of venous thrombi. Complications of DVT include pulmonary embolism and venous ulceration, and insufficiency. Approximately 200,000 deaths per year in the United States are attributable to pulmonary embolism secondary to DVTs.

21 **DEEP VENOUS THROMBOSIS**

ID/CC	A 25-year-old white female **continues to bleed** steadily after a normal, spontaneous vaginal delivery.
HPI	Manual exploration of the uterus reveals retained placental tissue that requires dilatation and curettage; 30 minutes after the procedure, the patient begins to **bleed profusely from her gums** and continues to bleed vaginally.
PE	Diffuse bleeding in gums and oral mucosa; **bleeding diathesis of skin** (both petechiae and purpura) with **oozing from venipuncture sites**.
Labs	Low fibrinogen. CBC: low platelet count. Prolonged PT and activated PTT; elevated fibrin split products, especially D-dimers.
Gross Pathology	May see complications such as renal cortical necrosis, limb thrombosis with gangrene, and ischemic adrenal necrosis.
Micro Pathology	**Microthrombi** in arterioles and capillaries, leading to **microinfarcts** in practically any organ; also **hemorrhages** and petechiae in involved organs.
Treatment	Treat underlying disorder; fresh frozen plasma; fibrinogen cryoprecipitate; platelets; aminocaproic acid with heparin.
Discussion	Disseminated intravascular coagulation (DIC) is a bleeding disorder that is due to consumption of platelets, fibrin, and coagulation factors secondary to excessive clotting in microcirculation. It is precipitated by **cancer, gram-negative septicemia, burns**, multiple **trauma**, and **obstetric complications**.

ID/CC   A **35-year-old man** complains of **pain in his calf muscles while walking** that is **relieved by rest** (INTERMITTENT CLAUDICATION) together with exertional chest pain.

HPI   He has a family history of **premature atherosclerotic coronary artery disease (CAD)**.

PE   VS: mild hypertension. PE: **obese; palmar xanthomas** and tendon xanthomas; **orange-yellow discoloration of palmar creases** (pathognomonic for **dysbetalipoproteinemia**); **tuboeruptive xanthomas** on pressure sites (elbows, buttocks, and knees); weak peripheral pulses.

Labs   LFTs normal; lipid profile reveals **elevated total cholesterol, triglycerides, and VLDL and reduced LDL and HDL**; chylomicron remnants present in fasting plasma; electrophoresis reveals **beta migrating VLDL**; isoelectric focusing shows **EII/EII genotype** (nearly pathognomonic).

Imaging   Angio, coronary: atherosclerotic coronary artery disease confirmed.

Gross Pathology   Yellowish intraluminal atherosclerotic plaques seen in the aorta and other large vessels.

Micro Pathology   Characteristic atherosclerotic plaques.

Treatment   **Weight reduction** to ideal body weight, regular exercise, **avoidance** of alcohol and other triglyceride-raising drugs; low-fat, low-cholesterol **diet**; in resistant cases, **gemfibrozil, high-dose nicotinic acid (niacin), and HMG-CoA reductase** inhibitors (statin drugs) may be used.

Discussion   Dysbetalipoproteinemia (TYPE III HYPERLIPOPROTEINEMIA) is defined as the presence of **VLDL particles that migrate to the** beta **position on electrophoresis** (normal VLDL particles typically migrate to the pre-beta location). Beta-VLDL particles are chylomicrons and VLDL remnants **caused in part by a mutant apo E** that impairs the hepatic uptake of apoprotein-E-containing lipoproteins (VLDL and chylomicrons).

ID/CC	A 61-year-old **white male** presents with marked **weakness, gingival bleeding**, and an **abdominal mass**.
HPI	He has a history of **recurrent bacterial infections** and has not traveled outside the United States.
PE	**Pallor; marked splenomegaly**; mild hepatomegaly; no lymphadenopathy, icterus, or ascites.
Labs	CBC/PBS: **anemia; decreased WBCs and platelets** (PANCYTOPENIA); **lymphocytes with characteristic long, thin cytoplasmic projections** ("HAIRY CELLS").
Imaging	CXR: normal. CT/US, abdomen: massive splenomegaly; mild hepatomegaly; no lymphadenopathy; no evidence of portal hypertension.
Gross Pathology	Liver, spleen, and bone marrow infiltrated by leukemic cells; splenomegaly may be significant.
Micro Pathology	**Bone marrow largely replaced by leukemic cells** (MYELOPHTHISIC BONE MARROW); large proportion are hairy cells and contain tartrate-resistant acid phosphatase (**TRAP**); splenic biopsy reveals leukemic infiltration of red pulp by hairy cells.
Treatment	Deoxycoformycin and α-interferon are highly effective; splenectomy.
Discussion	Hairy cell leukemia is a chronic **B-cell** malignancy; autoimmune syndromes are frequently seen, including vasculitis and arthritis. It is also characterized by **atypical mycobacterial infections**.
Atlas Link	UCV1 H-P2-024

HAIRY CELL LEUKEMIA

ID/CC An **8-year-old** white male presents with an erythematous skin **rash over the buttocks and legs** coupled with **joint pains, abdominal pain**, and **hematuria**.

HPI Three days before he had complained of cough, coryza, low-grade fever, and sore throat. He has a **history of allergy** to dust and pollen.

PE VS: hypertension. PE: **palpable purpuric skin lesions** over buttocks and legs; painful restriction of knee and ankle joint movement with swelling.

Labs CBC: **normal platelet count**; normal coagulation tests. Increased ESR; increased BUN and serum creatinine. UA: **RBCs and RBC casts** on urinary sediment. Positive stool guaiac test (due to occult blood).

Gross Pathology Necrotizing vasculitis of kidneys and lungs.

Micro Pathology Renal biopsy shows focal and segmental glomerulonephritis with crescents (mesangioproliferative); **mesangial IgA deposits** on immunofluorescence.

Treatment Supportive; steroids; high-dose immunoglobulin therapy experimental.

Discussion Henoch-Schönlein purpura is a generally self-limited, idiopathic disorder that is also known as anaphylactoid or vascular purpura; it is a **common vasculitis** (small vessel) **in children**.

Atlas Links 󰄱󰄲󰄳󰄴󰄵 PED-019A, PED-019B

HENOCH-SCHÖNLEIN PURPURA

ID/CC	A **6-year-old male** is brought to a specialist by his parents due to persistent **pain and tenderness on the right side of his chest** of a few months' duration.
HPI	There is **no history of trauma** to the affected area. The child is otherwise well and is growing normally.
PE	Exquisitely tender site found overlying fourth rib on right side anteriorly; remainder of exam unremarkable.
Labs	Routine lab parameters normal.
Imaging	CXR: **punched-out lesion** in fourth rib on right side.
Gross Pathology	**Intramedullary expanding, eroding lesion**.
Micro Pathology	Brownish granulation tissue containing **abundant foamy** histiocytes and **eosinophils** with leukocytes and giant cells.
Treatment	Lesions resolve spontaneously; surgical curettage may accelerate healing.
Discussion	Eosinophilic granuloma is a type of Langerhans cell histiocytosis; it is an indolent disorder that affects children and young adults, especially males. Solitary bone lesions may be asymptomatic or may cause pain and tenderness and, in some instances, pathologic fracture, but without any systemic manifestations. Diagnosis is based on radiographic demonstration of a localized destructive lesion arising from inside the marrow cavity. The **skull, mandible**, and **spine** are common locations. In some cases there may be spontaneous healing or fibrosis within a period of 1 to 2 years. The disease may also be multifocal, involving the lung, liver, spleen, or other organs.

ID/CC A 2-year-old boy is brought in for a pediatric consultation because his parents are concerned about **the child's protruding eyes** (EXOPHTHALMOS) and **excessive urine volume** (POLYURIA).

HPI The parents also state that the child has been febrile and has had multiple ear infections.

PE Low weight for age; bilateral exophthalmos; **painful swellings over head** (due to cystic bony lesions); no icterus; no lymphadenopathy; mild hepatosplenomegaly.

Labs CBC: normal blood counts. **Increased serum osmolality; decreased urine osmolality**.

Imaging XR, skull: **multiple rounded lytic lesions**.

Micro Pathology Bone biopsy from skull lesions show granulomatous lesions and characteristic Langerhans cells with coffee-bean-shaped nuclei and pale, abundant cytoplasm; **tennis-racket-shaped tubular structures** (BIRBEÇK GRANULES) on electron microscopy; positive S-100 protein and CD1 antigen.

Treatment Combination chemotherapy, curettage of bony lesions.

Discussion A type of **Langerhan's cell histiocytosis**, Hand–Schüller–Christian syndrome is multifocal, producing **diabetes insipidus** due to the involvement of the hypothalamus and exophthalmos from orbital infiltration by histiocytes.

ID/CC A **2-year-old** white male child is seen with complaints of **fever** followed by a **diffuse skin rash**.

HPI The child was apparently well a month ago, born after an uncomplicated pregnancy and delivery.

PE VS: tachycardia; fever. PE: mild pallor; otoscopy of left ear reveals dull, poorly mobile tympanic membrane with pus behind it (OTITIS MEDIA); generalized lymphadenopathy; hepatosplenomegaly; diffuse maculopapular eczematous rash.

Labs CBC: anemia; thrombocytopenia with leukopenia (PANCYTOPENIA); relative eosinophilia.

Imaging CT, abdomen: hepatosplenomegaly. XR: **cystic, rarefied lesions on skull and pelvis**.

Gross Pathology Skin shows presence of extensive **eczematoid rash**; large destructive bone lesions found on skull and pelvis.

Micro Pathology **Eosinophilic granulomatous lesions** in all involved organs; EM shows typical **Langerhans cells with characteristic Birbeck granules**; these cells were further found to be HLA-DR-positive and expressing **CD1 antigen**.

Treatment Corticosteroids; chemotherapy; surgery or radiotherapy for localized bone disease.

Discussion Letterer–Siwe disease is an acute or subacute clinical syndrome of unknown etiology affecting children less than 3 years old. It is marked by fever due to localized infection followed by a diffuse maculopapular eczematous purpuric skin rash and subsequent hepatosplenomegaly and generalized lymphadenopathy. It shows similarities to acute leukemia and other infectious processes. Diabetes insipidus, exophthalmos, and bone lesions are usually seen in combination.

ID/CC	A **24-year-old** white **male** complains of rapid enlargement of his abdomen, producing a dragging sensation, along with a **painless lump in his neck** for the past 2 months.
HPI	The patient also complains of intermittent **fever**, drenching **night sweats**, pruritus, and **significant weight loss**.
PE	Pallor; **unilateral nontender, rubbery, enlarged cervical lymph nodes; splenomegaly**; no enlargement of tonsils.
Labs	CBC/PBS: neutrophilic leukocytosis with lymphopenia; normocytic anemia. Elevated ESR; elevated serum copper and ferritin; negative Mantoux test.
Imaging	CXR: **bilateral hilar lymphadenopathy**.
Gross Pathology	Involved lymph nodes are rubbery and have **"cut-potato"** appearance of cut surface.
Micro Pathology	Lymph node biopsy shows large histiocyte cells with multilobed nuclei and eosinophilic nucleolus resembling **owl's eyes** (REED-STERNBERG CELLS); no bone marrow involvement on bone marrow biopsy.
Treatment	Radiotherapy and chemotherapy.
Discussion	Four patterns of Hodgkin's disease are seen on lymph node biopsy: lymphocytic predominance 5% to 10%; nodular sclerosis 65% to 75% (seen frequently in young women); mixed cellularity 20% to 30%; and lymphocyte depleted 10%. Prognosis worsens in this order. **Ann Arbor staging** I–IV with subclassification A (no constitutional symptoms) and B (weight loss, fever, night sweats) most accurately predicts prognosis. The disease **spreads to contiguous lymph nodes** before hematogenous dissemination.
Atlas Links	UCV1 H-P2-029 UCV2 IMI-049

ID/CC	A **3-year-old** white female is brought to the emergency room with a skin rash and **severe epistaxis**.
HPI	The patient had a **URI** consisting of a severe cough and a runny nose 10 days **before the onset of her symptoms**. She has no prior history of **prolonged bleeding** following minimal trauma.
PE	**Mucosal petechiae**; epistaxis; **hemorrhagic bullae** in buccal mucosa; spleen nonpalpable.
Labs	CBC: mild anemia; **low platelet count** (10,000); **RBCs and WBCs normal**. Prolonged bleeding time; normal PTT; normal PT.
Gross Pathology	**Purpura** (due to extravasation of blood from intravascular space into skin); pin-sized hemorrhages (PETECHIAE); ecchymosis (larger than purpura).
Micro Pathology	Normal bone marrow aspirate with **increased number of megakaryocytes**.
Treatment	Prednisone; splenectomy; IVIG.
Discussion	Idiopathic thrombocytopenic purpura (ITP) is an **autoimmune** disease with formation of **IgG antiplatelet antibodies** and subsequent platelet destruction in the spleen. It often **follows a viral infection** and is self-limited in children but chronic in adults.
Atlas Link	UCV2 PED-020

ID/CC	A **64-year-old black** male suffers from **bone pain**, weight loss, and **easy fatigability**.
HPI	He also complains of **recurrent URIs** and frequent nosebleeds.
PE	Pallor; **bone tenderness** in lower back and ribs; petechiae on buccal mucosa; no hepatosplenomegaly.
Labs	CBC/PBS: **normocytic, normochromic anemia**; neutropenia; **rouleau formation** (RBCs adhering together like stack of poker chips). **Elevated serum calcium**; normal alkaline phosphatase; markedly **increased ESR; gamma spike on serum protein electrophoresis** (**monoclonal** gammopathy). UA: **Bence Jones proteinuria** (due to IgG light chains).
Imaging	XR, plain: **punched-out, lytic bone lesions** in vertebrae, long bones, and skull (axial skeleton).
Gross Pathology	Multifocal replacement of normal bone tissue with tumor cells (plasmacytoma); pelvis, skull, and spine most affected.
Micro Pathology	Infiltration of bone marrow by normal-looking plasma cells (abundant cytoplasm, eccentric nuclei) in aggregates; **amyloid deposits** in kidney with renal tubular cast formation and interstitial fibrosis (can cause **renal insufficiency**); bone erosion and destruction of cortical bone.
Treatment	Chemotherapeutic regimen; hydration; treat hypercalcemia and hyperuricemia. Consider palliative radiation therapy.
Discussion	Multiple myeloma is a **primary malignancy of plasma cells** with replacement of normal bone marrow; it is the most common primary bone cancer. The prognosis worsens with anemia, renal failure, and multiple lytic lesions.
Atlas Links	▨◰◲◱ **H-P2-031A, H-P2-031B**

MULTIPLE MYELOMA

ID/CC	A 54-year-old white male complains of **easy fatigability**, shortness of breath, headache, and lightheadedness over the course of almost one year, with increasing severity.
HPI	He has also noticed a feeling of heaviness in his abdomen and **increasing girth** as well as recurrent deep pain in the legs and occasionally in the upper abdomen.
PE	**Massive splenomegaly**; enlarged liver; moderate amount of ascitic fluid; multiple petechiae on thorax and extremities; **no lymphadenopathy** (one differential feature shared with chronic myelogenous leukemia).
Labs	CBC/PBS: anemia (Hb 7.2); **low hematocrit**; anemia; immature WBCs and normoblasts seen simultaneously (LEUKOERYTHROBLASTIC SMEAR); **teardrop-shaped RBCs**; giant abnormal platelets.
Imaging	XR, plain: dense bones (generalized osteosclerosis).
Gross Pathology	**Extramedullary hematopoiesis**, which is prominent in liver and spleen, with significant increase in size and weight together with firm consistency.
Micro Pathology	**"Dry tap"** on **bone marrow** biopsy; hypocellular bone marrow (hypercellular early in disease); significant increase in number of megakaryocytes; replacement of marrow tissue with fibrosis (positive reticulin on silver stain); preservation of normal architecture of spleen.
Treatment	Transfusions; androgens; α-interferon; splenectomy.
Discussion	Also called agnogenic myeloid metaplasia, myelofibrosis with myeloid metaplasia is an idiopathic condition in which increased secretion of platelet-derived growth factor (PDGF) and TGF-β causes **replacement of bone marrow tissue with fibrosis**.
Atlas Links	⬛U̲C̲V̲1̲ H-P2-032A, H-P2-032B

MYELOFIBROSIS WITH MYELOID METAPLASIA

ID/CC	A 53-year-old white male notices **painless lumps** bilaterally **in his neck** that have slowly enlarged over the past 3 months.
HPI	Although he denies any pain, he admits to having episodes of mild **fever, night sweats**, and some **weight loss** over this period.
PE	Bilateral cervical **firm lymphadenopathy**; pallor; splenomegaly.
Labs	CBC: Coombs-positive hemolytic **anemia**; thrombocytopenia. **Elevated serum LDH** (a useful prognostic marker); hypogamma-globulinemia.
Imaging	CT/US: lymphadenopathy; splenomegaly.
Gross Pathology	Lymph nodes have grayish hue on outside and **"cut-potato"** appearance of cut surface.
Micro Pathology	Lymph node biopsy demonstrates nodular (well-differentiated) or diffuse-type (poorly differentiated) lymphocytic lymphoma; histiocytic and stem cell lymphoma.
Treatment	Alkylating agents in various combinations; radiotherapy if localized; bone marrow transplantation.
Discussion	Primary malignant neoplasms of lymphocytes arise in lymphoid tissue anywhere in the body; they occur mainly in lymph nodes but may involve intra-abdominal organs and bone marrow. The prognosis is more dependent on grade than on stage. Follicular (B-cell) lymphomas are the most common form and are associated with t(14;18) of bcl-2 (an anti-apoptosis protein). HIV patients have a higher incidence of non-Hodgkin's lymphoma.

NON-HODGKIN'S LYMPHOMA

ID/CC   A 62-year-old Jewish **male** visits his family doctor because of **epistaxis**, headache, and dizziness.

HPI   The patient had **black, tarry stools** (MELENA) 2 months ago and was previously admitted to the hospital for **deep venous thrombosis**. He also describes episodes of severe generalized **itching** (PRURITUS), primarily after showering.

PE   VS: **hypertension** (BP 170/100). PE: obese and **plethoric**; mild cyanosis; engorged, tortuous retinal veins with dark red hue on funduscopy; **palpable spleen**.

Labs   CBC: **markedly increased RBC count, hemoglobin level, and hematocrit**; WBCs and platelets also increased. Normal Po_2, Pco_2, and PT; increased vitamin B_{12} levels; increased leukocyte alkaline phosphatase; increased serum and urine uric acid levels; **decreased erythropoietin level** (distinguishes polycythemia vera from secondary polycythemia).

Gross Pathology   **Increased blood volume and viscosity** (RBC **sludging** and thrombus formation mainly in heart and brain); subnormal platelet function (bleeding tendency); increased frequency of peptic ulceration.

Micro Pathology   Bone marrow biopsy shows **increase in erythroid series precursors** and, to a lesser extent, in megakaryocytes and WBC precursors; thrombus formation with microinfarcts in brain and heart; myelofibrosis may ensue with characteristic findings.

Treatment   **Phlebotomy**; hydroxyurea; treat hyperuricemia.

Discussion   Polycythemia is characterized by an increase in RBC mass with increased blood volume and viscosity; it may be primary (polycythemia vera) or secondary (due to COPD, smoking, obesity, etc.). PCV may progress to chronic myelogenous leukemia, myelofibrosis, or acute myelogenous leukemia.

Atlas Link   ⬛UCV2⬛ IM1-052

ID/CC	A 4-year-old female is brought by her mother to the pediatric clinic after she finds **blood and a "lump" in the child's vagina**.
HPI	The child's father died of brain cancer, and her mother is receiving treatment for breast cancer. Her grandfather died of metastatic colorectal cancer.
PE	Pelvic exam reveals **ulcerated, polypoid, grape-like mass** arising from wall of vagina.
Labs	Routine lab work on urine, blood, and stool yields no pathologic findings.
Gross Pathology	Bulky tumor mass with multilobed papillary projections resembling mass of grapes.
Micro Pathology	Biopsy of tumor mass shows **desmin- and myoglobin-positive** (muscle tumor), elongated rhabdomyoblasts with large eosinophilic cytoplasm and **cross-striations**.
Treatment	Surgical resection with adjuvant chemotherapy, radiotherapy.
Discussion	Sarcoma botryoides is a polypoidal subtype of **embryonal rhabdomyosarcoma** that characteristically protrudes like a mass of grapes from the vagina or bladder; it is the most common sarcoma in children. Rhabdomyosarcomas are often found in **"cancer families"** (e.g., Li–Fraumeni syndrome).

ID/CC   A **10-year-old black child** presents with a chronic **nonhealing ulcer** on his lower leg.

HPI   He has had recurrent episodes of **abdominal and chest pain** (due to microvascular occlusion) along with **diminution of vision**. His maternal cousin suffers from a blood disorder.

PE   VS: fever. PS: **pallor; mild icterus**; funduscopy reveals **hypoxic spots with neovascularization** ("SEA FANS"); nonhealing chronic ulcer on left lower leg.

Labs   CBC/PBS: decreased hematocrit; megaloblastic anemia; **sickle-shaped RBCs; Howell–Jolly bodies and Cabot rings; sickling of RBCs** on sodium metabisulfite peripheral film (Sickledex prep). Serum bilirubin moderately elevated; quantitative hemoglobin electrophoresis shows **85% HbS**. UA: microscopic hematuria.

Imaging   CT/US, abdomen: **small, calcified spleen**.

Treatment   Local therapy for leg ulcer; laser therapy for proliferative retinopathy; antibiotic prophylaxis against capsulated bacteria; **hydroxyurea** may help increase fetal hemoglobin levels.

Discussion   Sickle cell anemia is caused by a **point mutation** on the gene coding for the β chain of hemoglobin; it shows **autosomal-recessive inheritance**. Glutamic acid is substituted by valine at position 6, leading to chronic hemolytic anemia. In the reduced form, HbS forms polymers that damage the RBC membrane. Factors that hasten sickling include acidosis and hypoxemia. Prenatal diagnosis is available for at-risk fetuses.

Atlas Links   UCV1 **H-P2-036, PM-P2-036**

ID/CC	An 11-month-old male presents with marked **pallor, failure to thrive, and delayed developmental motor milestones**.
HPI	The child's parents are **Indian** immigrants.
PE	Marked pallor; mild icterus; frontal bossing and **maxillary hypertrophy** ("CHIPMUNK FACIES"); **splenomegaly**.
Labs	CBC: severe microcytic, hypochromic anemia with **anisopoikilocytosis**; decreased reticulocytosis. **HbA absent; HbF 95%**; mildly increased unconjugated bilirubin.
Imaging	XR, skull (lateral): maxillary overgrowth and widening of diploic spaces with **"hair on end" appearance** of frontal bone, caused by vertical trabeculae.
Gross Pathology	Expansion of hematopoietic bone marrow, causing thinning of cortical bone or new bone formation.
Micro Pathology	Red marrow increased; yellow marrow decreased; marked erythroid hyperplasia in marrow (ineffective erythropoiesis).
Treatment	**Blood transfusion, folic acid supplement, iron chelation therapy** with desferrioxamine to reverse hemosiderosis, and **bone marrow transplantation** using HLA-matched sibling donors.
Discussion	Beta-thalassemia results from decreased synthesis of β-globin chains due to errors in the transcription, splicing or translation of mRNA. Alpha-thalassemia results from decreased synthesis of α-globin chains due to deletion of one or more of the four α genes that are normally present.

THALASSEMIA—BETA

ID/CC	A 23-year-old white **female** diagnosed 2 years ago as **HIV positive** is brought to the emergency room by her husband because of tachycardia, shortness of breath, headache, **intermittent disorientation**, and aphasia.
HPI	She had started prophylactic **TMP-SMX** 3 weeks ago. On the previous day, she had finished her menstrual period, which was abundant and had lasted for 7 days. Her husband also points out a **generalized red rash** all over her body.
PE	VS: tachycardia; **fever**. PE: pale skin and mucous membranes; **confusion** and apathy **with lucid periods; petechiae** on chest and extremities; positive Babinski's sign.
Labs	CBC/PBS: **microangiopathic hemolytic anemia** (Hb 7.2) with striking **reticulocytosis** and **fragmented RBCs** (SCHISTOCYTES); **low platelet count** (50,000); negative Coombs' test. Elevated indirect bilirubin (3.5). UA: hematuria. **Absent haptoglobin** (due to intravascular hemolysis); **normal coagulation tests; elevated LDH**.
Gross Pathology	Thrombus formation in several organs with platelet depletion and microangiopathic hemolytic anemia; kidney, brain, and heart most affected by thrombosis.
Micro Pathology	Multiple hyaline thrombi in brain, myocardium, renal cortex, adrenals, and pancreas.
Treatment	Plasmapheresis and fresh frozen plasma exchange; prednisone; splenectomy.
Discussion	Also known as Moschcowitz's syndrome, thrombotic thrombocy-topenic purpura (TTP) is an idiopathic disease found in **pregnant** and **HIV-positive** patients and following exposure to drugs such as **antibiotics** and **estrogens**.

ID/CC	An 18-year-old hospitalized male complains of **fever, nausea, vomiting**, and chest pain following a blood transfusion.
HPI	He was involved in a motorcycle accident and was rushed to the emergency room, where he **received five units of blood** before being taken to the OR for repair of a ruptured spleen and liver.
PE	VS: **fever**. PS: no hepatosplenomegaly or lymphadenopathy; surgical laparotomy wound unremarkable.
Labs	**Positive Coombs' test** (indicating autoantibodies to RBCs); decreased serum haptoglobin; elevated indirect bilirubin; **cola-colored urine** (due to hemoglobinuria).
Treatment	Hydration; force diuresis with mannitol or furosemide; hydrocortisone; alkalinize urine with HCO_3.
Discussion	Acute hemolytic transfusion reaction may be the result of complete complement activation; most commonly it is a result of **mismatched blood**, producing **intravascular hemolysis**. If severe, renal shutdown or disseminated intravascular coagulation (DIC) may occur.

TRANSFUSION REACTION—ACUTE HEMOLYTIC

ID/CC **During the administration of a blood transfusion,** a 45-year-old male presents with **fever, headache, and facial flushing**.

HPI An hour later he develops **frank rigors**. He has received **several transfusions in the past,** all of which were uneventful. The last one was **a few weeks ago**.

PE VS: fever; BP normal; tachycardia. PE: marked pallor; facial flushing; no cyanosis, icterus, or respiratory distress evident.

Labs CBC/PBS: **negative direct and indirect Coombs' test**. Normal serum bilirubin; no incompatibility found on repeat cross-matching of donor serum and patient's blood.

Treatment Supportive; antipyretics; **leukocyte-deplete future transfusions** by filtration.

Discussion Febrile nonhemolytic transfusion reaction is caused by **preformed leukoagglutinins** (cytotoxic antibodies) developed after previous transfusions; it is primarily a **type II hypersensitivity reaction**. Skin rash and pruritus or anaphylaxis occur in allergic reactions mediated by IgE (due to a **type I hypersensitivity reaction**).

ID/CC A 12-year-old white female is brought to the emergency room because of **uncontrollable bleeding following a tooth extraction**.

HPI She has a **history of prolonged bleeding** following minimal trauma. Her **father** also has a **bleeding disorder**.

PE Mucosal petechiae; epistaxis.

Labs **Prolonged bleeding time**; moderately **prolonged PTT; quantitative assay for factor VIII reduced**; platelets do not aggregate with ristocetin test; low von Willebrand's factor (vWF) antigen levels; low vWF activity.

Treatment Desmopressin, virally attenuated vWF concentrate (Humate-P); avoid aspirin.

Discussion A common congenital disorder of hemostasis, von Willebrand's disease is also called vascular hemophilia. Types I and II are **autosomal dominant**; vWF factor is necessary for platelet adhesion.

ID/CC	A **68-year-old** white male visits his doctor complaining of **weight loss**, increasing **fatigue, weakness**, headache, and **visual disturbances** over the past several months.
HPI	He also complains of **easy bruising** and **bleeding gums** while brushing his teeth.
PE	Generalized **lymphadenopathy; engorgement of retinal veins** with hemorrhages; moderate hepatosplenomegaly.
Labs	CBC/PBS: **anemia** (Hb 7.3); RBC **rouleau formation. IgM paraprotein** (monoclonal spike on serum protein electrophoresis); increased serum viscosity. UA: normal.
Imaging	XR, plain: **absence of lytic lesions** (vs. multiple myeloma).
Micro Pathology	Lymph node biopsy may be labeled pleomorphic lymphoma; bone marrow and spleen typically infiltrated with plasma cell precursors (plasmacytic lymphocytes); may show cytoplasmic eosinophilic, PAS-positive inclusion bodies (DUTCHER BODIES).
Treatment	Plasmapheresis; chlorambucil; cyclophosphamide.
Discussion	Waldenström's macroglobulinemia is a malignant B-lymphocyte disorder characterized by **excessive IgM** (macroglobulin) **production** and **hyperviscosity syndrome**.

ID/CC	A 2-year-old **male** is brought to his pediatrician because of recurrent **epistaxis** and chronic **eczematous dermatitis**.
HPI	He has a history of **recurring pneumonia** and bilateral **chronic suppurative otitis media**. A **male cousin** suffers from a **similar illness**.
PE	Epistaxis; eczematous dermatitis over both legs; several **purpuric patches** over skin; mild splenomegaly and cervical lymphadenopathy.
Labs	CBC/PBS: **thrombocytopenia**; lymphopenia. Decreased isohemagglutinins; decreased IgM; increased IgE, normal IgG, and increased IgA; **inability to form IgM antibody to carbohydrate antigens** (i.e., capsular polysaccharides of bacteria).
Treatment	Largely supportive; bone marrow transplant; splenectomy.
Discussion	Wiskott–Aldrich syndrome is a rare **X-linked recessive** disease with **B- and T-cell deficiency** characterized by a **triad of thrombocytopenia, eczema, and recurrent pyogenic infections**; it is due to a deletion of the WASP gene in the p11 region of the X chromosome. The condition is associated with an increased incidence of **lymphomas**.

WISKOTT–ALDRICH SYNDROME

ID/CC   A 6-year-old white female is brought to the emergency room by her mother because of severe **itching, joint pain**, and a **generalized skin eruption**.

HPI   She had received an **injection of penicillin 6 days before** for streptococcal tonsillitis. Her mother denies any relevant past medical history, including allergies. Once in the hospital, the child developed fever, **edema** of the ankles and knees, hematuria, and lethargy.

PE   VS: fever. PE: generalized **urticarial skin rash**; axillary and inguinal lymphadenopathy; splenomegaly; redness and swelling of knees and ankles.

Labs   Increased ESR; decreased C3, C4 levels. UA: proteinuria; hematuria.

Gross Pathology   Generalized wheals throughout body.

Micro Pathology   Vascular lesions show fibrinoid necrosis and a neutrophilic infiltrate; **immune complex deposition in kidney and joints**.

Treatment   Antihistamines; corticosteroids; aspirin; epinephrine if severe.

Discussion   Serum sickness is a **type III hypersensitivity reaction** (immune complex disease) with a latency period between exposure to the offending agent (drugs, serum) and the appearance of signs and symptoms; it is usually self-limiting.

ID/CC   A 50-year-old male presents with complaints of **palpitations** and **chest pain**.

HPI   The pain increases with physical activity and is relieved by rest. He has **multiple sexual partners**.

PE   VS: high-volume, **collapsing pulse** (WATER-HAMMER PULSE); **wide pulse pressure**. PE: pistol shots heard over brachial artery; to-and-fro murmur heard over femoral artery (DUROZIEZ'S MURMUR); cardiomegaly; loud aortic component of S2; grade III **early diastolic murmur** heard radiating down right sternal edge (murmur of aortic incompetence); mid-diastolic murmur heard at apex (AUSTIN FLINT MURMUR).

Labs   ECG: **left ventricular hypertrophy** with strain pattern. **VDRL and FTA-ABS positive**.

Imaging   CXR: **"tree bark" calcification** of ascending aorta and arch of aorta; **mediastinal widening and cardiomegaly**. Echo: **aortic incompetence**; left ventricular hypertrophy and dilatation.

Gross Pathology   Gross cardiac hypertrophy (cor bovinum); **aortic aneurysm** involving the **arch** and the **ascending aorta** and extending into the aortic valve, rendering it incompetent.

Micro Pathology   **Obliterative endarteritis** of vasa vasorum; degeneration and fibrosis of outer two-thirds of aortic media; compensatory irregular fibrous thickening of aortic intima.

Treatment   Penicillin; surgical excision and repair.

Discussion   Aortitis occurs in the **tertiary stage of syphilis**, often arising many decades after the primary infection. Weakening of the aortic wall causes dilatation of the aortic root as well as aortic incompetence and aneurysms. Intimal fibrosis causes narrowing of the openings of the coronary arteries (ostial stenosis), resulting in myocardial ischemia.

Atlas Link   [UCV1] PG-P2-045

INFECTIOUS DISEASE

ID/CC A term female newborn is noted to have **edema, dyspnea, cyanosis, and marked jaundice**.

HPI Her **mother is blood type** AB **Rh-negative**. Her **previous childbirth** was an uneventful full-term vaginal delivery conducted outside the United States 4 years ago. The mother **did not receive any subsequent immunizations**.

PE Pallor; **marked jaundice**; hypotonia; **S3 and S4**; hepatosplenomegaly; **generalized edema**.

Labs Blood type of **mother** AB **Rh negative**; blood type of father A Rh positive; **blood type of first child** A **Rh positive**. Mother's serum: **positive** indirect **Coombs' test**, anti-D antibody titer > 1:64. Neonate's serum: positive direct Coombs' test, increased indirect bilirubin.

Gross Pathology Brain specimen from autopsy reveals yellow staining of basal ganglia by unconjugated bilirubin (KERNICTERUS).

Treatment Phototherapy (promotes elimination of bilirubin); exchange transfusion.

Discussion The mother produced anti-D (IgG) antibodies owing to her exposure to D antigen during her delivery of an Rh-positive infant. In her subsequent pregnancy, these antibodies crossed the placenta and reacted with the fetus's RBCs (Rh positive), producing hemolysis and **fetal heart failure with generalized edema** (HYDROPS FETALIS). To prevent Rh isoimmunization, all Rh-negative mothers with an Rh-positive fetus should receive **RhO (D) immune globulin** following deliveries, abortions, ectopic pregnancies, or even amniocentesis.

ERYTHROBLASTOSIS FETALIS

ID/CC	Paramedics are called at 7:00 a.m. because a **2-month-old male**, the child of Cuban immigrants, cannot be awakened by his mother; upon arrival, it is clear that the child has been dead for at least 4 hours.
HPI	The child was slightly premature, but aside from this, his history was unremarkable. There was nothing that could directly explain the episode. On directed history, **the mother admits to being a smoker and remembers that the child had a URI 4 days ago**.
PE	No pathologic cause revealed that could explain death.
Gross Pathology	Autopsy reveals petechiae on pleural and pericardial surfaces, pulmonary congestion, and scattered foci of lymphocytic tissue in interstitium of lungs.
Discussion	Sudden infant death syndrome (SIDS) refers to **death of an infant under 1 year** of age, usually during sleep, in which **death remains unexplained** even after complete autopsy; most have a history of minor URIs.

SUDDEN INFANT DEATH SYNDROME (SIDS)

ID/CC	A 17-year-old white male undergoing chemotherapy for disseminated Hodgkin's lymphoma complains of severe headaches, nausea, and weight loss.
HPI	The patient had been on **aminoglycosides**. When questioned, he is uncertain of place and time, but despite his confusion he describes his urine as appearing reddish-orange over the past few weeks.
PE	Confused but alert; underweight; no acute distress.
Labs	Lytes: increased potassium. UA: **oliguria**; hematuria; mild proteinuria; granular casts in urine; renal tubular epithelial cells in sediment; isotonic urine osmolality; **elevated urinary sodium** (> 40 mEq/L). Increased serum inorganic phosphorus; **azotemia** with BUN/creatinine ratio of 5 (within normal limits).
Gross Pathology	Kidneys enlarged, flabby, and pale with edema.
Micro Pathology	Necrosis of tubular epithelial cells that slough into lumen, forming casts and causing blockade; hydropic degeneration of epithelium.
Treatment	Discontinue offending agent; fluid and electrolyte management.
Discussion	Acute tubular necrosis is defined as acute tubular damage resulting in acute renal failure; it is caused by prolonged ischemia or toxins (nephrotoxic drugs) and is usually reversible.
Atlas Links	UCVI PM-P2-048, PG-P2-048

ID/CC	A 47-year-old white male enters the emergency room complaining of a sudden-onset, **severe headache** that is the **"worst headache of his life."**
HPI	He also describes slow-onset dull pain in his left flank and blood in his urine. He was recently treated for **recurrent UTIs**, which were attributed to an enlarged prostate gland. His **father** died of **chronic renal failure**, and his paternal **grandfather** died of **cerebral hemorrhage**.
PE	VS: hypertension (BP 170/110). PE: palpable, nontender **abdominal mass** on both flanks; nuchal rigidity.
Labs	UA: albuminuria; microscopic **hematuria** (no WBCs or casts). Slightly increased BUN, creatinine.
Imaging	Angio, neuro: ruptured **berry aneurysm**. CT/US, abdomen: **multiple kidney and liver cysts**.
Gross Pathology	Kidneys markedly enlarged and heavy with hundreds of cysts that almost replace normal parenchyma; cysts thick-walled, ranging from a few millimeters to several centimeters in diameter.
Micro Pathology	Cystic dilatation of tubules; epithelial cell hyperplasia; cuboidal epithelium lining cysts.
Treatment	Dialysis and renal transplantation.
Discussion	Adult polycystic kidney disease (APKD) is an **autosomal-dominant** disease caused by a defect in **chromosome 16** in which the renal parenchyma is converted to hundreds of fluid-filled cysts, resulting in progressive renal failure in adulthood. Cysts may also involve the pancreas, liver, lungs, and spleen. It is associated with berry aneurysms of the circle of Willis, hypertension, and mitral valve prolapse.

ADULT POLYCYSTIC KIDNEY DISEASE (APKD)

ID/CC	A 5-year-old **female** is brought to the pediatrician because her mother noticed **blood in her urine** and **diminished vision acuity**.
HPI	Her family is **Mormon**. Her mother suffers from chronic renal failure.
PE	VS: BP normal. PE: appears well nourished; bilateral **sensorineural hearing loss**; bilateral **cataracts**.
Labs	CBC/PBS: normochromic, normocytic **anemia**. High-tone sensorineural loss detected on audiometry; elevated serum creatinine and BUN. UA: **proteinuria; hematuria**; RBC casts.
Gross Pathology	Small, smooth kidneys.
Micro Pathology	Longitudinal thinning and splitting of glomerular basement membrane, producing characteristic laminated appearance with glomerular sclerosis; interstitial infiltrate containing fat-filled macrophages (LARGE FOAM CELLS).
Treatment	ACE inhibitors; renal transplantation.
Discussion	Alport's syndrome can be autosomal-dominant or x-linked and is caused by a defect in the α chain of type IV collagen. It is also called hereditary chronic nephritis and is progressive in males.

ALPORT'S DISEASE

ID/CC	A 45-year-old white female complains of palpitations and shortness of breath, morning swelling of the eyes, arms, and legs, and numbness of the lower legs together with weight loss and fatigue.
HPI	Her past medical history is unremarkable.
PE	Mild cardiomegaly; **macroglossia**; pitting **edema** in lower extremities; **ascites; cardiac arrhythmia** on auscultation.
Labs	UA: proteinuria. ECG: ventricular hypertrophy and low voltage **(restrictive cardiomyopathy)**. Hypoproteinemia; hyperlipidemia.
Imaging	CXR: biventricular cardiac enlargement.
Gross Pathology	Pathologic deposition of amyloid glycoprotein in several organs, primarily heart, kidney, and rectal and gingival tissue; kidneys pale, waxy, gray, and firm; spleen and liver may be enlarged; deep-brown discoloration characteristic of amyloid-infiltrated organs exposed to iodine.
Micro Pathology	**Apple-green birefringence** in polarized light when stained **with Congo red**; amyloid deposition in mesangium as well as in endothelium surrounding hepatic sinusoids and in spleen; hyaline thickening of arteriolar walls, leading to narrowing of lumen and ischemia.
Treatment	Supportive.
Discussion	Primary amyloidosis commonly presents with nephrotic syndrome. Amyloidosis may be primary (in which the proteins are monoclonal **immunoglobulin light chain**) or secondary to chronic inflammatory states (especially rheumatoid arthritis and tuberculosis). The primary type is often associated with B-cell dyscrasias, especially **multiple myeloma**, and in these cases **Bence Jones proteins** are almost always present in the serum and urine.
Atlas Link	UCV1 PM-P2-051

AMYLOIDOSIS—PRIMARY

ID/CC	A 56-year-old male complains of **urinary frequency** and interruption of the urinary stream over the past 6 months; he also complains of having to wake up multiple times during the night to urinate (NOCTURIA).
HPI	The patient's history includes one episode of acute urinary retention one month ago that was relieved with catheterization. He denies any history of hematuria (vs. carcinoma of the bladder) or back pain (vs. metastasized prostatic carcinoma). He also admits to having a **reduced caliber of urine stream** and **terminal dribbling** as well as **urinary hesitancy**.
PE	Digital rectal exam reveals **smooth enlargement of the prostate** protruding into the rectum; overlying rectal mucosa mobile; **bladder percussible up to umbilicus**.
Labs	UA: 2+ bacteria; positive nitrite and leukocyte esterase. Prostate-specific antigen (PSA) levels normal; urodynamic studies demonstrate **bladder neck obstruction** with increased residual urine volume; mildly elevated serum creatinine and BUN.
Imaging	US: benign-appearing enlargement of median lobe.
Gross Pathology	Enlarged prostate with well-demarcated nodules up to 1 cm in diameter in **median lobe** of prostate.
Micro Pathology	Both stroma and glands show **hyperplasia** on biopsy; fibromyoadenomatous hyperplasia seen in which proliferating glands are surrounded by proliferating smooth muscle cells and fibroblasts.
Treatment	Finasteride; transurethral resection of prostate (TURP). Treat associated UTIs with appropriate antibiotics (e.g., TMP-SMX, ciprofloxacin).
Discussion	Age-dependent changes of estrogens and androgens are believed to cause benign prostatic hypertrophy (BPH); an increasing incidence is noted starting at 40 years of age. It affects up to 75% of men by the age of 80 years.
Atlas Link	UCVI PG-P2-052

ID/CC	A 65-year-old **white male** complains of **painless hematuria** of several days' duration.
HPI	He is a **heavy smoker**.
PE	Lungs clear; abdomen nontender; no palpable masses; genitalia within normal limits; no lymphadenopathy.
Labs	CBC: slight normocytic, normochromic anemia. UA: **hematuria** and abundant epithelial cells.
Imaging	IVP/Cystogram: **irregular filling defects** above trigone.
Gross Pathology	Nodular, **cauliflower-like** lesion with central necrosis and minimal invasion of bladder wall.
Micro Pathology	Cytology of urine shows malignant cells. Biopsy of bladder shows grade I, stage B **transitional cell carcinoma** (TCC) arising from uroepithelium and projecting into bladder.
Treatment	Surgery (transurethral resection); radiotherapy; chemotherapy.
Discussion	There is a threefold increase in risk in men, and the average age at diagnosis is 65. Risk factors for papillary carcinoma of the bladder include industrial exposure to **arylamines** (especially 2-naphthylamine), **cigarette smoke,** *Schistosoma haematobium* infection (although most *Schistosoma* infections are associated with squamous neoplasia), **analgesic abuse** (especially phenacetin), and long-term **cyclophosphamide** therapy. Complications include invasion of perivesicular tissue, ureteral invasion with urinary obstruction (leading to hydronephrosis, pyelonephritis, and renal failure), and metastases to the lung, bone, and liver. TCC appears to be associated with mutations in the p53 tumor suppressor gene and deletions in chromosomes 9p and 9q.
Atlas Link	UCVI PM-P2-053

BLADDER CANCER

ID/CC	A 65-year-old male presents with **acute urinary retention**.
HPI	For the past few years, he has noted an **increased frequency** of micturition along with increased **hesitancy, urgency**, decreased force and stream of urine, and a feeling of **incomplete evacuation** of the bladder. For the past few months he has begun to experience **increasing fatigability and lassitude**.
PE	Pallor; bladder full on abdominal examination; rectal exam reveals **grade III prostate enlargement**.
Labs	CBC: normocytic anemia. Lytes: hypocalcemia; hyperphosphatemia. **Elevated BUN and creatinine**. UA: proteinuria; **no RBCs or casts seen**.
Imaging	US, kidneys: **bilateral hydroureter and hydronephrosis**.
Micro Pathology	In addition to hydronephrosis and hydroureter, interstitial kidney disease is seen on microscopic examination.
Treatment	**Transurethral resection** of the prostate (TURP) to relieve the obstruction is the basic and most useful step.
Discussion	Obstructive nephropathy results from the **impaired outflow of urine** but may also **produce chronic interstitial damage**. Obstructive nephropathy is common in childhood (from congenital abnormalities) and in individuals older than 60 years, when benign prostatic hypertrophy and prostatic and gynecologic cancers become more common.

ID/CC	A 48-year-old white female is admitted to the hospital because of worsening **generalized edema** and weakness along with **hypertension**.
HPI	She has a long history of type I **diabetes mellitus** but no history of hematuria, recent sore throat, or skin infections.
PE	VS: **hypertension** (BP 160/110). PE: **generalized pitting edema**; no evidence of pleural effusion or ascites; lung bases clear on auscultation; JVP normal; neither kidney palpable; funduscopic exam reveals presence of **proliferative diabetic retinopathy**.
Labs	**Elevated** fasting **blood sugar** (234 mg/dL); elevated glycosylated hemoglobin (10%); **elevated BUN and serum creatinine; decreased serum albumin; elevated blood cholesterol**. UA: presence of sugar and **3+ protein**; broad casts and **fatty casts**; elevated quantitative protein (3.5 gm/24 hr).
Micro Pathology	**Increased mesangial matrix** on renal biopsy; **thickening of capillary basement membrane** combined with acellular eosinophilic nodules in mesangium (KIMMELSTIEL-WILSON DISEASE); hyaline arteriosclerosis of both afferent and efferent arterioles; no immune complex deposits seen.
Treatment	Blood sugar control; control of systemic hypertension, preferably with ACE inhibitor; dietary protein and phosphate restriction; avoidance of nephrotoxic drugs; dialysis or renal transplantation.
Discussion	Diabetic glomerulosclerosis is a renal manifestation of diabetic microangiopathy and presents at least 10 years after diabetes appears (more commonly in IDDM); it is usually the prelude to end-stage diabetic renal disease.
Atlas Link	UCVI PM-P2-055

ID/CC	A **36-year-old** white **male** complains of a chronic cough of several months' duration, accompanied by lightheadedness, fatigue, and malaise; yesterday he **coughed up blood**.
HPI	He also describes intermittent fever and headaches in addition to small volumes of **dark orange urine**. He denies alcohol use but admits to being a heavy **smoker**.
PE	Diffuse pulmonary crackles bilaterally.
Labs	Azotemia. UA: oliguria; **hematuria**; proteinuría. **Iron deficiency anemia**; blood detected in sputum. ABGs: hypoxemia.
Imaging	CXR: bilateral alveolar infiltrates.
Gross Pathology	Increase in weight of lungs with areas of necrosis; **kidneys** enlarged and pale with decreased consistency.
Micro Pathology	Kidney biopsy shows proliferative, necrotizing, **crescentic glomerulonephritis** with accumulation of neutrophils and macrophages in Bowman's capsule; characteristic **linear IgG deposits in glomerular basement membrane and alveolar septa** on immunofluorescence; **anti-glomerular basement membrane antibodies** in serum; necrotizing hemorrhagic **alveolitis** on lung biopsy.
Treatment	Plasma exchange; corticosteroids; immunosuppressive therapy.
Discussion	Goodpasture's syndrome is hemorrhagic alveolitis with nephritis and iron deficiency anemia caused by anti-glomerular basement membrane antibodies (type II hypersensitivity reaction).
Atlas Link	UCV1 PM-P2-056

ID/CC	A 45-year-old **black** male presents with uncontrolled **hypertension** and complains of severe occipital headache and ringing in his ears.
HPI	He also reports **markedly diminished urine output over the past 24 hours**. On directed questioning, he also reports **some visual blurring**.
PE	VS: **severe hypertension**. PE: funduscopy reveals presence of **papilledema** with **hypertensive retinopathy**.
Labs	UA: proteinuria; microscopic hematuria; **red cell casts. Elevated BUN and creatinine**. CBC: microangiopathic hemolytic anemia. ECG: left-axis deviation with left ventricular hypertrophy.
Imaging	Echo: concentric left ventricular hypertrophy with reduced ejection fraction. US, abdomen: presence of **parenchymal renal disease in normal-sized kidneys** (unlike that of benign nephrosclerosis, where there are bilateral contracted kidneys).
Micro Pathology	Pathologic changes include **fibrinoid necrosis of arterioles** (NECROTIZING ARTERIOLITIS), **hyperplastic arteriolosclerosis** ("ONION SKINNING"), and necrotizing glomerulitis associated with a thrombotic microangiopathy.
Treatment	**Reduction of diastolic blood pressure to at least 100 mmHg; maintain urine output > 20 mL/hour.**
Discussion	**Sodium nitroprusside** is the safest and most effective drug for use in hypertensive emergencies; because it does not impair myocardial blood flow, it is especially useful in underlying ischemic heart disease. However, it is metabolized to cyanide and thiocyanate; therefore, prolonged use may lead to cyanide toxicity or to thiocyanate toxicity. Blood thiocyanate levels should be determined frequently.

ID/CC	A 22-year-old white male complains of recurrent episodes of **"bloody urine"** that lasted for several days **in conjunction** with a **URI**.
HPI	He was well until the onset of symptoms.
PE	Pallor; slight palpebral edema.
Labs	UA: proteinuria; **red cell casts in urine**; gross hematuria. **Increased serum IgA.**
Micro Pathology	Focal glomerulonephritis involving only selected glomeruli with **mesangial proliferation** and segmental necrosis with crescents; immunofluorescence typically reveals mesangial **IgA deposits** with some IgM, IgG, and C3.
Treatment	Supportive; IgA deposits commonly reappear following kidney transplantation.
Discussion	IgA nephropathy is idiopathic but associated with upper respiratory or GI infections lacking a latency period (vs. poststreptococcal glomerulonephritis). Lesions are variable and may be mesangioproliferative, focal proliferative, or possibly crescentic glomerulonephritis. The glomerular pathology seen in Berger's disease is similar to that seen in **Henoch–Schönlein purpura**, which is seen in children. It is seen with increased frequency in patients with celiac disease and liver disease (due to defective IgA clearance). **Chronic renal failure may ultimately develop.**

ID/CC	A **30-year-old black woman** presents with **pain** in both her knee **joints** and in the small joints of the hand together with mild fever, anorexia, weight loss, and loss of hair.
HPI	She also has a history of **recurrent oral ulcerations** and a **photosensitive skin rash**. No joint deformities are reported.
PE	VS: hypertension. PE: oral **aphthous ulcers** noted; erythematous **photosensitive skin rash; "butterfly rash"** over malar area of face; pallor; no abdominal or renal bruits heard.
Labs	CBC: normocytic, normochromic **anemia**. UA: microscopic hematuria with **RBC casts** in addition to proteinuria. **Elevated BUN and creatinine; antinuclear antibodies positive** in high titer; **LE cell phenomenon** positive; **anti-Sm antibody and anti-ds DNA antibody positive; VDRL positive** but FTA-ABS negative.
Micro Pathology	Renal biopsy reveals features of **diffuse proliferative glomeru-lonephritis**. Electron microscopy reveals **immune complex deposits** that are typically **subendothelial** and form **"wire loops."**
Treatment	Corticosteroids; cytotoxic drugs (cyclophosphamide, azathio-prine, and chlorambucil); long-term hemodialysis or transplant.
Discussion	There are five patterns of lupus nephritis. Class I is normal by light, EM, and immunofluorescence microscopy. Class II presents as **mesangial lupus glomerulonephritis** and is found in about 25% of patients; it is associated with minimal hematuria or proteinuria. Class III is characterized by **focal proliferative** glomerulonephritis and is associated with recurrent hematuria and mild renal insufficiency. Class IV is described in this case and is by far the most common form. Class V presents as **membranous glomerulonephritis** and is seen in 15% of cases; it induces severe proteinuria or nephrotic syndrome.

LUPUS NEPHRITIS

ID/CC	An 11-year-old white girl is brought to the pediatrician because of headache, chest palpitations, and ringing in her ears together with **generalized edema**.
HPI	She has no history of dyspnea, sore throat, skin infections, or fever. Careful questioning reveals that she has also had **hematuria**.
PE	VS: hypertension (BP 140/100). PE: **generalized** (including periorbital) **pitting edema**; JVP normal; lung bases clear; neither kidney palpable; no evidence of pleural effusion or ascites.
Labs	Elevated BUN and serum creatinine; decreased serum albumin; elevated serum triglycerides; serum **hypocomplementemia**; antinuclear antibody (ANA) negative; normal ASO titers. UA: **fatty casts and oval bodies in addition to proteins**.
Micro Pathology	Diffuse glomerular involvement with thickened capillary walls and lobular mesangial proliferation on light microscopy. **Splitting of basement membrane causing railroad-track appearance** with PAS reagent or silver stain; **prominent granular immunofluorescence**; mesangial and subendothelial deposits of immune complexes.
Treatment	Corticosteroids; renal transplantation.
Discussion	Membranoproliferative glomerulonephritis (MPGN) is idiopathic but may be associated with inherited deficiencies of complement components and partial lipodystrophy. It is subdivided into two types: type I MPGN (both classic and alternative complement pathways activated) and type II MPGN (dense deposit disease; activation of alternate complement pathway). Approximately 50% of patients with MPGN will go on to develop **chronic renal failure**. There is a **high recurrence rate** following renal transplantation.

ID/CC	A 47-year-old black diabetic female complains of weight loss, progressive shortness of breath, and **swelling of the lower legs** and arms.
HPI	Her past medical history is unremarkable.
PE	Pallor; pitting edema in extremities; decreased lung sounds with crackles bilaterally in lower lung fields; **periorbital edema; ascites**.
Labs	UA: **proteinuria** (> 3.5 g/24 hr); lipiduria with oval fat bodies and fatty and waxy casts in urinary sediment. **Hypoalbuminemia** (< 3 g/dL); **hyperlipidemia** (serum cholesterol 250 mg/dL).
Gross Pathology	Kidneys enlarged, pale, and rubbery; renal vein thrombosis may be present.
Micro Pathology	**Thickened basement membrane**; subepithelial deposits of IgG and C3 along basement membrane seen in **"spike and dome"** pattern on methenamine silver stain; immune deposits in a **"lumpy-bumpy"** (discontinuous) pattern on immunofluorescence.
Treatment	Corticosteroids; cyclophosphamide; renal transplantation; ACE inhibitors reduce urinary protein loss.
Discussion	Nephrotic syndrome may be idiopathic or caused by membranous glomerulonephritis (the most common cause in adults), minimal change disease (LIPOID NEPHROSIS) (the most common in children), focal glomerulosclerosis, or membranoproliferative glomerulonephritis. Patients with nephrotic syndrome have **hypercoagulability** secondary to loss of antithrombin III in the urine (e.g., increased incidence of peripheral vein thrombosis).

61   **MEMBRANOUS GLOMERULONEPHRITIS (MPGN)**

ID/CC	A **5-year-old** white male presents with **generalized edema** and abdominal distention, producing respiratory embarrassment.
HPI	The child had a **URI** 1 week ago.
PE	VS: BP normal. PE: generalized pitting edema; free **ascitic fluid** in peritoneal cavity; shifting dullness and fluid thrill present; normal funduscopic exam.
Labs	UA: 4+ **proteinuria** (> 3 g/24 h). **Hypoalbuminemia; hypercholesterolemia**; hypertriglyceridemia; decreased serum ionic calcium; normal C3 levels; normal serum creatinine and BUN.
Gross Pathology	Kidneys slightly enlarged, soft, and yellowish.
Micro Pathology	Light microscopy and immunofluorescent studies **normal on renal biopsy** (no evidence of immune complex deposition). EM reveals uniform and diffuse loss of the podocytic foot processes.
Treatment	**Corticosteroids**; salt-restricted diet; diuretics; electrolyte therapy and monitoring.
Discussion	Also called **lipoid nephrosis**, minimal change disease is the most common cause of idiopathic **nephrotic syndrome in children** and is associated with infections or vaccinations. It carries a **good prognosis**.
Atlas Links	UCV1 **PM-P2-062** UCV2 IM2-036

ID/CC	A 68-year-old **black** male complains of **dysuria, progressively increased urinary frequency**, and **back pain** that has lasted several months.
HPI	He reports **high animal-fat intake**.
PE	Nodular, **rock-hard, irregular area of induration** in **peripheral lobe** of prostate on digital rectal exam; **midline furrow** between prostatic lobes **obscured; extension to seminal vesicles** detected.
Labs	Markedly elevated **prostate-specific antigen** (PSA) and **acid phosphatase**.
Imaging	Transrectal US, prostate: **hypoechoic masses** in peripheral zone with extension to seminal vesicles. Nuc, bone scan: **hot lesions of spine, sacrum, and pelvic bones** (axial skeleton). CT/MR: prostate mass with capsular penetration and enlarged seminal vesicles.
Gross Pathology	Irregularly enlarged, firm, nodular prostate.
Micro Pathology	Core needle biopsy of prostate reveals single layer of malignant neoplastic cells arranged haphazardly in adenoplastic stroma.
Treatment	Prostatectomy with radiation; orchiectomy; leuprolide; antiandrogens such as flutamide.
Discussion	A primary malignant neoplasm of the prostate commonly arising from the peripheral zone (70%), prostate carcinoma is the **most common male cancer**. Its prognosis and treatment depend heavily on stage. Most cases are diagnosed in **asymptomatic** men on digital rectal exam. Prostate cancer exhibits **hematogenous dissemination**, most commonly to **bone**, forming **osteoblastic lesions**. The tumor can also invade sacral nerve roots, causing significant pain.
Atlas Links	UCV1 PM-P2-063, PG-P2-063

PROSTATE CARCINOMA

ID/CC	A 60-year-old white male complains of right **flank pain** and **hematuria**.
HPI	He has been a **heavy smoker** for the past 24 years; he **lost 5 pounds over the past month** and is not on a diet.
PE	VS: low-grade fever; moderate hypertension. PE: pallor; **palpable mass** in right flank.
Labs	Elevated ESR. CBC/PBS: normocytic, normochromic **anemia**. UA: gross **hematuria**.
Imaging	IVP/CT/US: mass in upper pole of right kidney. MR: no invasion of renal vein or inferior vena cava (IVC).
Gross Pathology	Yellowish areas of necrotic tissue with focal areas of hemorrhage within renal parenchyma.
Micro Pathology	Polygonal **clear cells** (containing glycogen) with evidence of cytologic atypia invading renal parenchyma.
Treatment	Right **nephrectomy**; consider renal-sparing partial nephrectomy.
Discussion	The **most common renal tumor**, renal cell carcinoma is frequently sporadic but is seen in association with **von Hippel-Lindau syndrome** and dialysis-related **acquired polycystic kidney disease**. It frequently invades the **renal vein and IVC** and metastasizes to lungs and bone via hematogenous dissemination. It can also cause **paraneoplastic syndromes** (secondary to the production of erythropoietin, parathyroid-like hormone, ACTH, and renin).
Atlas Link	UCV1 PM-P2-064

ID/CC	A 63-year-old white male complains of **sudden-onset pain in** the right **flank** together with gross **hematuria**, nausea, and vomiting.
HPI	He is **overweight**, has been diabetic for 15 years, is a heavy **smoker** and drinker, and has been surgically treated for **aortofemoral occlusive disease** (graft).
PE	VS: no fever; mild hypertension (BP 150/100). PE: **acute distress**; pallor; sweating; severe right flank pain; **xanthelasma** in both eyelids.
Labs	Normal BUN and creatinine. UA: **hematuria**. ECG: old silent anterior wall myocardial infarction. Elevated **LDH**.
Imaging	CT, abdomen: **wedge-shaped, nonenhancing lesion in right kidney**. US, renal: edematous kidney with focal region of decreased color flow.
Gross Pathology	Pale, yellowish-white, wedge-shaped area with hemorrhagic necrosis in renal cortex.
Micro Pathology	Coagulation necrosis involving renal cortical nephrons extending into corticomedullary junction.
Treatment	Remove arterial obstruction by thrombolysis; heparin anticoagulation to prevent recurrence.
Discussion	Risk factors for embolic events include atherosclerosis and mural thrombi in the heart and aorta, infectious endocarditis vegetations, and atheromatous plaques in the aorta. Complications from renal artery embolism include renal failure, hypertension, acute pyelonephritis, and renal abscess.

ID/CC	A **30-year-old** white female is found to be **hypertensive** on routine physical exam.
HPI	She claims to have **no history of hypertension** and denies any changes in lifestyle or excessive stress.
PE	VS: **hypertension** (BP 175/105). PE: loud S2; funduscopic exam normal; **abdominal bruit** present.
Labs	**Elevated plasma renin**; hypokalemia.
Imaging	Angio, renal: confirmatory; unilateral left **renal artery stenosis in a "string of pearls" pattern**.
Gross Pathology	In fibromuscular dysplasia, the renal artery lumen is decreased due to hyperplastic fibrotic wall thickening.
Micro Pathology	Muscular hyperplasia with fibrosis and segmental stenosis.
Treatment	**ACE inhibitors** (contraindicated in bilateral renal artery stenosis). Balloon angioplasty; stenting; surgical correction.
Discussion	Renovascular hypertension is secondary systemic hypertension caused by hypersecretion of renin from hypoperfused kidney(s). It is most often caused by **fibromuscular dysplasia (young Caucasian women)** or **atherosclerosis (older men)** and accounts for < 5% of all causes of hypertension.
Atlas Link	UCV1 PG-P2-066

ID/CC	A **36-year-old** white male presents with **progressive painless enlargement of the left testicle** of 2 months' duration.
HPI	He also complains of a sense of heaviness in his scrotum. He denies any history of pain or trauma at the site.
PE	Walnut-sized, nontender, smooth, **firm mass at upper end of left testicle; mass does not transilluminate**; epididymis and vas deferens normal on palpation; prostate and seminal vesicles normal on digital rectal exam; abdominal lymph nodes not palpable; no hepatomegaly.
Labs	Normal levels of hCG; **normal levels of serum α-fetoprotein and LDH; histologic** diagnosis based on postoperative specimen study.
Imaging	CXR: no metastasis. US, abdomen and pelvis/scrotum: solid intratesticular mass. CT: no metastasis.
Gross Pathology	Solid white bulging mass within testis.
Micro Pathology	Sheets of germ cells containing clear cytoplasm with lymphocytes in fibrous stroma.
Treatment	Orchiectomy with retroperitoneal lymph node dissection; chemotherapy with cisplatin; radiotherapy.
Discussion	Seminoma is the most common type of germ cell tumor. Dysgerminomas in ovaries are histologically similar. Tumors are extremely **radiosensitive**. It is associated with a good prognosis. **Cryptorchidism** predisposes to the development of testicular tumors.
Atlas Links	**UCV1** PG-P2-067, PM-P2-067

ID/CC A 30-year-old man complains of a small **painless nodular swelling over his right testicle** that he noticed a few months ago, coupled with **increasing growth of his breast tissue**.

HPI He also complains of mild shortness of breath on exertion (DYSPNEA), cough, and blood-streaked sputum.

PE VS: normal. PE: bilateral gynecomastia (breast tissue palpable); small, **pea-shaped swelling** involving the **right testicle**; testicular sensation lost; no transillumination; **left supraclavicular lymphadenopathy**; hepatomegaly.

Labs CBC: mild anemia. Serum β-hCG elevated.

Imaging CXR: two "cannonball" parenchymal masses (due to metastases). CT, abdomen: enlarged retroperitoneal lymph nodes and multiple hepatic metastases. US, scrotum: complex, solid right testicular mass.

Gross Pathology Small, pea-shaped hemorrhagic mass seen in right testicle.

Micro Pathology Polygonal, comparatively uniform **cytotrophoblastic cells** with clear cytoplasm growing in sheets and cords, mixed with **multinucleate syncytiotrophoblastic cells** that have **eosinophilic vacuolated cytoplasm** with readily **demonstrable hCG**; no well-developed villi seen.

Treatment **Chemotherapy** with **cisplatin, etoposide, and bleomycin** in some combination, followed by **radical inguinal orchiectomy** and **retroperitoneal lymph node dissection**; gynecomastia regresses once the source of hCG (the tumor) is removed.

Discussion **Choriocarcinoma** is the **most malignant** of all testicular tumors; it metastasizes relatively early via both the **lymphatics** and the **bloodstream** even when it remains very small locally. **Follow up with β-hCG levels**.

ID/CC	A newborn baby is evaluated for **ambiguous external genitalia**.
HPI	The baby was delivered vaginally at full term without any pre-, intra-, or postnatal complications; the mother did not take **hormones** or any other **drugs during pregnancy**.
PE	**Incompletely virilized external genitalia**; hypospadias; **bilateral inguinal swelling**.
Labs	Karyotype: **46,XY. Müllerian structures absent**; inguinal swellings proved to be **maldescended dysgenetic testes**.
Imaging	US: absence of müllerian structures and presence of dysgenic testes.
Micro Pathology	Testes characterized by **seminiferous tubule degeneration** and invasion by connective tissue arranged in whorls.
Treatment	**Gonadectomy** to protect against increased risk of testicular tumor; **hormone replacement** therapy given at puberty.
Discussion	The incidence of **gonadal tumors in dysgenetic gonads** may reach up to 30%, making orchiectomy and subsequent hormone replacement the best therapeutic option.

ID/CC	A 23-year-old **white** male is seen by his family physician because of **dyspnea**, **bilateral enlargement of the breasts** (GYNECOMASTIA), and a **painless lump in the right testis** of approximately 2 months' duration.
HPI	He denies any history of STDs, genital ulcers, drug use, or trauma.
PE	Bilateral nontender gynecomastia (due to increased hCG); left supraclavicular lymphadenopathy; 5-cm **hard mass** palpable **on right testis**, distorted shape; normal rectal exam.
Labs	**Markedly elevated blood hCG and α-fetoprotein (AFP).**
Imaging	US/MR, testes: **solid intratesticular mass** with some foci of hemorrhage (intratesticular masses usually malignant).
Micro Pathology	Cytotrophoblastic and syncytiotrophoblastic cells with hCG demonstrable within cytoplasm.
Treatment	High radical inguinal orchiectomy followed by cisplatin-based combination chemotherapy.
Discussion	Testicular cancer may be pure or mixed (mixed germ cell neoplasm) and is highly malignant with early and widespread metastasis. It is the most common neoplasm in men aged 20 to 35. Yolk sac tumors produce only AFP, whereas choriocarcinomas produce only hCG.

ID/CC	A 9-year-old black male is brought into the emergency room because of **sudden-onset** severe **pain** that he experienced in the lower abdomen and **scrotum** while playing soccer.
HPI	He has no relevant medical history. Upon admission, he became nauseated and vomited three times.
PE	Irritability; right **testicle tender, swollen**, and elevated; palpable normal epididymis anteriorly; **increased pain with elevation of mass** (PREHN'S SIGN); no hernia palpable; no transillumination of mass.
Labs	UA: mild leukocytosis.
Imaging	US, scrotum: asymmetric decreased color flow in testicle. Nuc-Tc99: **doughnut sign** (due to central testicular ischemia and circumferential collateral flow).
Gross Pathology	Testicle markedly enlarged with hemorrhagic necrosis; scrotum may be purplish; cord twisted.
Micro Pathology	Severe venous congestion; interstitial hemorrhage; hemorrhagic necrosis.
Treatment	**Immediate surgery** (detorsion and fixation of testis to scrotum) due to risk of testicle loss (less than 4 hours); contralateral orchiopexy prophylactically (high incidence of bilaterality); atrophic testicle should be removed due to possible autoimmune destruction of contralateral testis.
Discussion	Testicular torsion is a surgical emergency that needs to be differentiated from orchitis, epididymitis, and strangulated hernia. It is seen more frequently in an **undescended testicle** (CRYPTORCHIDISM).

TESTICULAR TORSION

ID/CC	A 45-year-old man with a high-grade **non-Hodgkin's lymphoma** develops **oliguria, severe malaise, and fatigue** 36 hours following **chemotherapy treatment**.
PE	Carpopedal **spasm** present; neither kidney is palpable; urinary bladder is empty.
Labs	Lytes: hyperkalemia, **hyperuricemia**, and hyperphosphatemia with secondary hypocalcemia. **BUN and creatinine elevated**. UA: acidic urine with numerous **rhomboid crystals**; no casts or cells seen.
Treatment	Maintenance of good hydration, brisk alkaline diuresis, and **pretreatment with allopurinol** are keys to prevention of this syndrome; once acute renal failure has developed, fluid and electrolyte balance must be maintained and dialysis may be necessary.
Discussion	Tumor lysis syndrome is most often seen in patients with **lymphoma or leukemia** but is also seen in patients with a variety of solid tumors. The presence of a **large tumor burden, a high growth fraction, an increased pretreatment LDH level and uric acid level**, or preexisting renal insufficiency increases the likelihood that a patient will develop tumor lysis syndrome. Increased levels of uric acid, xanthine, and phosphate may result in precipitation of these substances in the kidney. Renal sludging and acute renal insufficiency or failure further aggravate the metabolic abnormality.

ID/CC	A **3-year-old** male is brought to his pediatrician for evaluation of an **abdominal mass** that his parents noticed.
HPI	The child has been well all his life.
PE	Slight pallor; weight and height within normal range; nontender, large, firm, and smooth intra-abdominal mass to right of midline; right **cryptorchidism** and **aniridia**.
Labs	UA: microscopic **hematuria**; normal urinary vanillylmandelic acid (VMA); BUN increased; serum erythropoietin elevated.
Imaging	IVP: displacement and distortion of right pelvicaliceal system. CT, abdomen: tumor arising from right kidney with areas of low density (due to necrosis); persistent ellipsoid area of enhancement (due to compressed renal parenchyma); no evidence of vascular invasion.
Gross Pathology	Whitish, solid tumor with areas of hemorrhagic necrosis distorting normal renal parenchyma compressed into narrow rim; may be involvement of perirenal fat; metastasis usually to lungs.
Micro Pathology	Glomeruloid and tubular structures enclosed within spindle cell stroma; areas of cartilage, bone, or striated muscle tissue.
Treatment	Surgical removal of kidney containing tumor; chemotherapy with actinomycin D and vincristine; radiotherapy.
Discussion	Nephroblastoma (WILMS' TUMOR) is a malignant tumor of embryonal origin. It is associated with deletions on **chromosome 11p** involving the WT-1 gene and should be differentiated from neuroblastoma and malignant lymphoma, which are other small cell tumors of childhood. **WAGR syndrome** consists of Wilms' tumor, aniridia, genitourinary abnormalities, and mental retardation.

ID/CC	A 45-year-old white female is rushed to the OR because of **shock** due to postoperative bleeding; during intubation, she **vomits and aspirates** that day's breakfast.
HPI	She had undergone a cholecystectomy 2 days before and had presented with postoperative bleeding requiring surgical exploration.
PE	VS: **tachycardia; tachypnea; fever; hypotension**. PE: **central cyanosis**; warm, moist skin; **intercostal retraction; inspiratory crepitant rales** heard over both lung fields.
Labs	CBC/PBS: marked **leukocytosis** with neutrophilia; fragmented RBCs; thrombocytopenia. ABGs: **severe hypoxemia with no improvement on 100% oxygen**. Increased BUN and creatinine; increased AST and ALT.
Imaging	CXR: typical **diffuse and symmetric parahilar ("bat-wing" pattern) alveolar filling** process suggestive of **noncardiogenic pulmonary edema**.
Gross Pathology	Formation of **hyaline membranes** with proteinaceous deposits in alveoli; **pulmonary edema** with red, heavy lungs which, combined with **widespread atelectasis**, produce **stiff lung** with fibrosis.
Micro Pathology	Endothelial and alveolocapillary damage with edema, hyaline membrane formation, and inflammatory infiltrate; **loss of surfactant** with fibroblast activity in later stages.
Treatment	Mechanical ventilation, antibiotics, steroids, close monitoring of hemodynamic function.
Discussion	Adult respiratory distress syndrome is a condition that is associated with **high mortality**; it is caused by gram-negative **sepsis, massive trauma**; burns, disseminated intravascular coagulation (DIC), acute pancreatitis, narcotic overdose, and near-drowning. It is characterized by diffuse alveolar capillary injury, which leads to an increase in vascular permeability and pulmonary edema.
Atlas Link	UCVT1 PM-P2-074

ID/CC A **65-year-old male** presents with **progressively increasing cough and dyspnea** on exertion.

HPI He is a **retired construction worker** and has a nearly **100-pack-year smoking** history.

PE VS: normal. PE: grade II **clubbing**; fine crackles auscultated bilaterally over lung bases.

Labs CBC: normal. PFTs: mixed obstructive and restrictive disease pattern; reduced DL_{CO}. Microscopic exam of sputum reveals **golden-brown beaded rods** (ASBESTOS BODIES) composed of asbestos fibers coated with an iron-containing proteinaceous material.

Imaging CXR: irregular linear, **interstitial infiltrates** in lower lobes with circumscribed radiopaque densities (PLEURAL PLAQUES). CT (high resolution): posterior and lateral pleura thickened with **calcified plaques** seen bilaterally.

Gross Pathology Diffuse pulmonary **interstitial fibrosis** with **bilateral pleural calcification** and thickening and involvement of the diaphragm.

Micro Pathology Calcium-containing dense pleural opacities and plaques of collagen; asbestos bodies.

Treatment Supportive and symptomatic treatment (oxygen, bronchodilators, antibiotics); **prevention of further exposure**; **smoking cessation**; counseling regarding **high risk** of **bronchogenic carcinoma** and **malignant mesothelioma**.

Discussion Prolonged exposure to asbestos in significantly cumulative doses results in **pulmonary parenchymal scarring**. This process is self-perpetuating, but cessation of exposure may slow disease progression. Complications include **bronchogenic carcinoma, malignant mesothelioma, cor pulmonale**, and death.

ID/CC	A 10-year-old girl is brought into the ER in **acute respiratory distress**.
HPI	The patient is known to be **allergic** to cats and pollen; her mother states that she had a **recent URI**. She also complains of a history of moderate **intermittent dyspnea that is exacerbated by exercise**.
PE	VS: no fever; **tachypnea** (RR 32); BP: normal. PE: inspiratory and **expiratory wheezes** (due to bronchoconstriction, small airway inflammation); boggy and pale nasal mucosa; **accessory muscle use during breathing**; enlarged chest AP diameter; **hyperresonant** to percussion.
Labs	ABGs: primary respiratory alkalosis (hyperventilation). CBC: **eosinophilia** (13%). PFTs: low FEV_1/FVC.
Imaging	CXR: hyperinflation with flattened diaphragms (increased residual volume due to **air trapping**); peribronchial cuffing.
Gross Pathology	**Hyperinflation** with air trapping in alveoli; **plugs of inspissated mucus**; edema of mucosal lining.
Micro Pathology	Inflammatory infiltrate of bronchial epithelium, mainly eosinophilic; plugging of airways **with thickened mucus** (CURSCHMANN'S SPIRALS); hypertrophy of mucous glands; elongated rhomboid crystals derived from eosinophil cytoplasm (CHARCOT–LEYDEN CRYSTALS); hyperplasia of smooth muscle of bronchi.
Treatment	Inhaled, oral, and parenteral bronchodilators; steroids; cromolyn; zafirlukast.
Discussion	Bronchial asthma is characterized by **hyperreactivity of the airways** and obstruction due to bronchospasm, edema, and mucus. It is also known as **reactive airway disease**.

ID/CC   A 50-year-old white male develops a **fever 24 hours after surgery**.

HPI   He underwent an emergency **laparotomy** for a perforated peptic ulcer without any intraoperative or immediate postoperative complications.

PE   VS: fever; BP normal; **tachypnea; tachycardia**. PE: no cyanosis; **scattered rales** and **decreased breath sounds**; no calf tenderness; no hematoma or discharge from wound; no inflammation of IV line veins; no urinary symptoms.

Labs   ABGs: mild **hypoxemia**. CBC: slight neutrophilic leukocytosis. Blood and sputum culture sterile. ECG: sinus tachycardia.

Imaging   CXR: **dense opacity in right lower lobe** (collapsed lobe) with elevation of right hemidiaphragm (due to volume loss).

Treatment   Chest physiotherapy (incentive spirometry); deep inspirations; mucolytic agents.

Discussion   Postoperative atelectasis is the most common cause of postoperative fever in the first 48 hours; alveolar collapse is produced by occlusion due to viscid secretions favored by recumbency, hypoventilation, and oversedation. Other causes of postoperative fever, usually seen later in the postoperative period, include UTI, IV catheter infection, deep venous thrombosis, wound infection, and drug reactions.

ID/CC	A 14-year-old male presents with complaints of **exertional dyspnea, chronic productive cough**, and **occasional hemoptysis**.
HPI	He was diagnosed with **cystic fibrosis** at age 4 and has had **recurrent pulmonary infections** requiring frequent hospitalizations.
PE	VS: low-grade fever (38°C); tachycardia (HR 110); tachypnea (RR 28). PE: pallor and grade II **clubbing** noted; **coarse crackles** auscultated over both lung fields.
Labs	CBC: **normocytic, normochromic anemia**; low hematocrit. Sputum culture reveals *Staphylococcus aureus*. PFTs: decreased FEV_1/FVC suggestive of obstructive pathology.
Imaging	XR, chest: increased bronchovascular markings; honeycomb appearance (due to end-on shadows of dilated bronchioles); loss of lung volume (atelectasis). CT (high resolution), chest: **dilated bronchioles with "signet ring" appearance** (due to adjacent branch of pulmonary artery).
Gross Pathology	Long, tubelike, irreversibly dilated bronchioles extending to the pleura with loss of lung parenchyma.
Treatment	**Supportive measures; antibiotics; bronchodilators**, expectorants, and **physical therapy** to promote bronchial drainage. Surgery may be indicated for localized or segmental bronchiectasis or when medical therapy fails.
Discussion	Dilatation of the bronchial tree leads to infections and to further irreversible dilatation. Underlying causes include **obstruction** due to tumor, foreign bodies, and mucus impaction; **congenital disorders** such as Kartagener's syndrome, Williams-Campbell syndrome, and **cystic fibrosis**; and **infections** due to *Bordetella pertussis*, togavirus, RSV, measles, and *Mycobacterium tuberculosis*. **Complications** include **lung abscesses, metastatic brain abscesses, amyloidosis, and cor pulmonale**.

ID/CC	A **60-year-old male** is referred to an allergist for late-onset **asthma** that has been **unresponsive to bronchodilators and antibiotics**.
HPI	He has also been having chest pain (ANGINA), fatigue, anorexia, and pain in both calves (CLAUDICATION) on exertion that are of recent onset.
PE	VS: tachypnea; mild fever; **mild hypertension** (BP 150/100) (secondary to renal vascular involvement). PE: marked respiratory distress; widespread **wheezes** bilaterally; numerous **purpuric lesions on feet** (due to cutaneous small vessel vasculitis).
Labs	CBC: mild anemia; leukocytosis (> 10,000/μL); Hct < 35%; thrombocytosis (> 400,000/μL); **eosinophilia (> 1000/μL)**. **Elevated BUN and creatinine**; P-ANCA positive. UA: **proteinuria**; presence of **RBCs**, WBCs, and **granular casts**. PFTs: FEV_1/FVC ratio reduced (**obstructive pulmonary disease**). ECG: sinus tachycardia.
Imaging	CXR: **bilateral upper and lower lobe infiltrates** and noncavitating nodules.
Gross Pathology	Lung shows hemorrhagic infarcts secondary to thrombi in affected arteries.
Micro Pathology	Transbronchial lung biopsy shows **granulomatous lesions in vascular and extravascular sites accompanied by intense eosinophilia**; skin biopsy of purpuric lesions shows **vasculitic lesions**—fibrinoid necrosis of media with mixture of inflammatory cells extending along adventitia; occasional aneurysms and secondary thromboses seen; the arterial internal elastic lamina is destroyed and intima and media are thickened.
Treatment	**Prednisolone** effective in inducing remission; **cyclophosphamide** used in those **refractory** to steroids; monitor disease course using **ESR levels**.
Discussion	Churg–Strauss syndrome is an idiopathic systemic **small- and medium-vessel granulomatous vasculitis** (grouped with polyarteritis nodosa [PAN], which does not involve lungs) that is characterized by a triad of late-onset **asthma**, a fluctuating **eosinophilia**, and an **extrapulmonary vasculitis**.

CHURG–STRAUSS SYNDROME

ID/CC	A 50-year-old white male **smoker** presents with **productive cough, copious sputum**, shortness of breath, and **fever**.
HPI	The patient has a **40-pack-year** smoking history. He has also experienced chronic dyspnea on exertion; chronic **productive cough**, usually **in the mornings**, for several years; and multiple colds each winter.
PE	VS: fever. PE: stocky build with plethora; wheezes.
Labs	CBC: elevated WBC count (14,000); neutrophils predominant; **secondary polycythemia**. *Streptococcus pneumoniae* or *Haemophilus influenzae* on Gram stain of sputum sample. ABGs: decreased Po_2; elevated Pco_2. PFTs: decreased vital capacity; **decreased FEV_1**.
Imaging	CXR: increased bronchovascular markings in lower lung fields.
Gross Pathology	Thick mucous secretion; edema of bronchial mucosa.
Micro Pathology	**Increased size and number of mucous glands** (Reid's index > 50); inflammation; fibrosis; squamous metaplasia.
Treatment	Antibiotics; bronchodilators; smoking cessation.

ID/CC A 55-year-old male complains of progressively increasing **shortness of breath on exertion** for the past few months.

HPI He also complains of a nonproductive mild cough and has a **40-pack-year smoking history** but has no history of hemoptysis or occupational exposure to inorganic or organic dusts.

PE VS: moderate tachypnea. PE: moderate respiratory distress; **using accessory muscles of respiration**; fullness of neck veins during expiration; chest **barrel-shaped; percussion note hyperresonant; cardiac and liver dullness** are **obliterated**; scattered rhonchi bilaterally; **heart sounds heard distant** but normal.

Labs ABGs: mild hypoxia with respiratory alkalosis. PFTs: increased residual volume; **decreased FEV$_1$/FVC ratio** (OBSTRUCTIVE DISEASE PATTERN); decreased DL$_{CO}$.

Imaging CXR, (PA view): **hyperlucent** lung fields with a few **bullae**; flattening of diaphragm and elongated tubular heart shadow.

Gross Pathology Air spaces dilated; **upper lobes most affected**.

Micro Pathology Pattern of **centrilobular emphysema**: alveolar septa are visibly diminished in number along with increased air spaces.

Treatment Cessation of smoking, bronchodilators, steroids in resistant cases, antibiotics during acute exacerbations, and home oxygen therapy.

Discussion Emphysema is defined as abnormal permanent enlargement of the air spaces distal to the terminal bronchiole accompanied by the destruction of the alveolar walls; emphysema may involve the acinus and the lobule uniformly in a pattern called panacinar, or it may primarily involve the respiratory bronchioles, termed centriacinar. Panacinar emphysema is common in patients with **α$_1$-antitrypsin deficiency**. Centriacinar emphysema is commonly found in cigarette smokers and is rare in nonsmokers; it is usually more extensive and severe in the upper lobes.

Atlas Links UCV1 PG-P2-081, PM-P2-081

ID/CC A 37-year-old **male** in the ICU develops **petechiae, altered sensorium, and marked dyspnea** that prove refractory to oxygen therapy.

HPI **Twenty-four hours ago**, he was admitted to the hospital with **fractures of the shafts of both femurs, the pelvis, and the right humerus**, sustained following a fall from a 20-foot-high stepladder.

PE VS: fever; marked dyspnea. PE: **delirium; central cyanosis**; using accessory muscles of respiration; wheezing heard over both lung fields.

Labs ABGs: **profound arterial hypoxemia with hypercapnia.** CBC/PBS: thrombocytopenia. **Fat demonstrated in urine and sputum**; normal PT and PTT.

Imaging CXR: early, normal; later, bilateral perihilar ("BAT-WING") appearance of **pulmonary infiltrates** without cardiomegaly (due to noncardiogenic pulmonary edema). XR, plain: long bone fractures.

Micro Pathology Obstruction of pulmonary vessels by fat globules; chemical pneumonitis.

Treatment Intermittent positive pressure ventilation with 100% oxygen, supportive management.

Discussion Fat embolization usually occurs **24 to 72 hours after fractures of the shafts of the long bones.**

Atlas Link UCV1 PM-P2-082

FAT EMBOLISM

ID/CC   A 50-year-old **farmer** presents with severe **shortness of breath** (DYSPNEA) and **fatigue**.

HPI   He also complains of a **dry cough** and **mild fever**. His symptoms are exacerbated when he works in the fields, especially when he comes into contact with **moldy hay**. He does not smoke and drinks alcohol occasionally.

PE   VS: tachycardia; tachypnea; mild fever. PE: moderate respiratory distress; scattered rhonchi and **bilateral fine rales**.

Labs   CBC: leukocytosis with shift to left. Elevated ESR; **serum antibodies against thermophilic *Actinomyces* organisms**; bronchoalveolar lavage shows marked lymphocytosis, primarily suppressor-cytotoxic T cells. PFTs: **restrictive lung disease** pattern.

Imaging   CXR: bilateral **reticulonodular infiltrates with fibrosis**. CT: areas of ground-glass abnormalities with centrilobular peribronchial nodules.

Gross Pathology   Fibrosis with honeycombing.

Micro Pathology   Bronchoscopic lung biopsy reveals interstitial pneumonia with lymphocytes and plasma cells in alveolar walls as well as scattered focal granulomas with foreign body giant cells.

Treatment   Strict avoidance of contact with aspergillus spores; steroids.

Discussion   Hypersensitivity pneumonitis (allergic alveolitis) refers to interstitial lung disease that results from inhalation of organic antigens. Hypersensitivity pneumonitis is believed to have an immunologic basis (e.g., cytotoxic, immune complex, and cell-mediated reactions); **the most common form of hypersensitivity pneumonitis, called farmer's lung, is caused by inhalation of a thermophilic *Actinomyces* organism present in moldy hay and grain**. Other common causes of hypersensitivity pneumonitis include pigeon breeder's disease and bird fancier's disease, in which inhaled serum proteins from pigeons or parakeets induce the syndrome. Humidifier lung disease results from exposure to contaminated forced-air systems.

HYPERSENSITIVITY PNEUMONITIS

ID/CC	A 65-year-old male complains of progressive shortness of breath on exertion and a chronic **dry cough**.
HPI	The patient has **never smoked** cigarettes and has no history of exposure to occupational dusts or fumes; he has not had a productive cough or hemoptysis.
PE	VS: warm but **cyanosed**; tachycardia (HR 108); tachypnea; BP normal. PE: **clubbing present**; JVP not elevated; heart sounds normal with no additional sounds or murmurs; respiratory examination reveals presence of bilateral **basal fine inspiratory crepitations**.
Labs	ABGs: hypoxemia. PFTs: **decreased DL$_{CO}$**; desaturation with exercise; proportionately reduced FEV$_1$ and FVC so that ratio remained unchanged (due to restrictive disease). Bronchoalveolar lavage predominantly neutrophilic; serum calcium and ACE levels low.
Imaging	CXR: reticulonodular shadows in both lower lung fields with occasional areas of **"honeycombing."** CT (high resolution): fibrosis in lower lung lobes suggestive of usual **interstitial pneumonitis pattern of IPF**.
Micro Pathology	Bronchoscopically obtained lung biopsy reveals presence of fibrosis, inflammatory round cell infiltrate, and thickening of the alveolar septa.
Treatment	Systemic steroids.
Discussion	The main differential diagnoses to consider are lung fibrosis associated with a connective tissue disorder (rule out by history and clinical exam), extrinsic alveolitis due to organic dusts, left-sided heart failure, sarcoidosis (rule out on the basis of absence of any other system involvement, normal calcium and ACE levels, negative Kveim's test, and lack of hilar lymphadenopathy observed on CXR), lymphangitis carcinomatosa (rule out on biopsy and CT), and pneumoconiosis. The onset of idiopathic pulmonary fibrosis is typically in the fifth or sixth decade.
Atlas Link	UCV1 PM-P2-084

ID/CC	A 58-year-old male presents with **shortness of breath** (DYSPNEA), **hoarseness, cough**, and **hemoptysis**.
HPI	He has an **80-pack-year smoking history**. Over the past 2 months, he has also had a **significant loss of appetite and weight**.
PE	Marked pallor; **cachexia; clubbing**; mild wheezing at rest; chest barrel shaped (emphysematous) and movements diminished on right; **dullness to percussion** over right middle lobe; **no breath sounds** heard over right middle lobe; vocal fremitus reduced in same area.
Labs	CBC: **normocytic, normochromic anemia**. Gram and ZN stains of sputum for acid-fast bacilli negative; sputum cytology reveals presence of **malignant squamous cells**.
Imaging	CXR/CT: irregular hilar mass on right side, producing an obstruction atelectasis of right middle lobe. Bronchoscopy: right-sided hilar mass obstructing right middle bronchus.
Gross Pathology	Postsurgical specimen reveals an irregular invasive mass of grayish-tan tumor spreading out from right middle bronchus and obstructing it.
Micro Pathology	Biopsy reveals presence of malignant squamous cells, cellular stratification, **intercellular bridges**, and **"keratin pearls."**
Treatment	Surgical resection can be potentially curative in patients with non-small-cell lung cancer.
Discussion	Lung cancer is the **most preventable cancer**. Owing to the increased incidence of smoking, lung cancer has exceeded breast cancer as the leading cause of cancer death in women. A **Pancoast's tumor** is a lung tumor located at the lung apex in the superior pulmonary sulcus that causes compression of the cervical sympathetic plexus, resulting in **Horner's syndrome** (ptosis, miosis, anhidrosis) as well as scapular pain and ulnar nerve radiculopathy.
Atlas Links	UCV1 PM-P2-085, PG-P2-085

ID/CC A 67-year-old male is referred to a clinic for evaluation of **pleuritic pain, weight loss**, gradually progressive **dyspnea**, and a **nonproductive cough** of a few months' duration.

HPI He worked in a **shipyard** for 20 years before retiring, an occupation that involved **asbestos exposure**.

PE VS: normal. PS: **clubbing of fingers**; mild cyanosis; **reduced chest expansion**; end-inspiratory rales auscultated over both lung fields; **dull percussion, reduced breath sounds**, and egophony in right side (due to pleural effusion).

Labs CBC/PBS: polycythemia; **marked eosinophilia**. PFTs: **restrictive pattern** observed (decreased vital capacity and decreased total lung capacity with normal FEV_1/FVC ratio). Reduced diffusion capacity; pleural effusion bloody and shows acidic pH (< 7.3).

Imaging CXR: right-sided pleural effusion; diffuse bilateral **interstitial fibrosis; parietal pleural calcifications**. CT: highly irregular pleural-based masses; hemorrhagic effusion.

Gross Pathology Thick, **fibrous pleural plaques with calcification**; diffuse interstitial fibrosis; asbestos compounds form nest for further deposition of iron salts and glycoproteins (FERRUGINOUS ASBESTOS BODIES).

Micro Pathology Epithelioid pattern of pleural malignant sarcomatous transformation with cellular atypia and high mitotic index.

Treatment Surgery; poor prognosis.

Discussion **Occupational exposure to asbestos** is found in 80% of cases of malignant mesothelioma; it produces **lung fibrosis** with a **restrictive pattern**. Asbestos and tobacco exposure synergistically increase the risk of lung adenocarcinoma.

Atlas Links UCV1 PG-P2-086, PM-P2-086

MALIGNANT MESOTHELIOMA

ID/CC A 37-year-old female comes to the emergency room complaining of **pleuritic pain** on the right side of her chest and **dyspnea** together with fever and a productive cough.

HPI There is no hemoptysis. The pain is typically **sharp and stabbing**, and it arises when she takes a deep breath (PLEURISY).

PE **Decreased chest movement during inhalation** on right side; **dullness** on percussion of right lung base; **reduced or absent breath sounds** over right lung base; bronchial breath sounds auscultated on right side; friction rub; location of **dullness moves with respiration; decreased tactile fremitus** over right lung.

Labs CBC: elevated WBC count with predominance of neutrophils. Gram-positive diplococci on sputum smear and culture; **elevated protein, decreased glucose, and many neutrophils in pleural exudate.**

Imaging CXR: consolidation of right lower lobe; pleural effusion on right side. XR, lateral decubitus: **layering of fluid** (therefore not loculated).

Treatment Antibiotics and needle drainage of effusion (THORACENTESIS); sometimes obliteration of pleural space.

Discussion Pleural effusions may be due to infection (viral, bacterial, mycobacterial, fungal); other causes are malignancies, congestive heart failure, cirrhosis, nephrotic syndrome, trauma, pancreatitis, collagen diseases, and drug reactions. Effusions may be **transudative** (< 3 g/dL of protein) or **exudative** (> 3 g/dL of protein). Elevated pleural fluid LDH levels may be suggestive of malignancy. **Transudative pleural effusions** are commonly caused by congestive heart failure, cirrhosis, and nephrotic syndrome, whereas **exudative pleural effusions** are caused by TB, infections, malignancy, pancreatitis, pulmonary embolus, and chylothorax (milky pleural fluid).

ID/CC   A 25-year-old white **male** complains of **sudden pleuritic chest pain** and **shortness of breath** that **awakens him at night**.

HPI   He **smokes** one pack of cigarettes a day and states that his paternal **uncle once had a similar episode**.

PE   **Tall, thin** patient; diaphoretic and feels weak; left chest expands poorly on inspiration; trachea and apex beat displaced to right; left side **hyperresonant** to percussion; **decreased breath sounds; decreased tactile fremitus**.

Labs   ABGs: decreased Po_2; elevated Pco_2.

Imaging   CXR: partial collapse of left lung with no lung markings except **thin line parallel to chest wall; costophrenic sulcus abnormally radiolucent** ("DEEP SULCUS" SIGN) in supine film.

Gross Pathology   Types: traumatic, spontaneous, tension, open; common causes: surgical puncture, rupture of emphysematous bullae, positive pressure mechanical ventilation, bronchopleural fistula.

Treatment   Pneumothorax evacuation via pleural catheter (CHEST TUBE).

Discussion   The usual cause of spontaneous pneumothorax is rupture of a **subpleural bleb**.

ID/CC	A 40-year-old male is brought to the ER with complaints of **sudden-onset, severe right-sided chest pain followed by severe difficulty breathing**.
HPI	He is a chronic smoker and has predominantly **emphysematous** COPD.
PE	VS: severe tachycardia; tachypnea; hypotension; no fever. PE: **cyanosis; trachea shifted** to left; chest exam reveals **hyperresonant percussion note on right, diminished breath sounds,** and **decreased tactile fremitus**.
Labs	ABGs: hypoxemia; respiratory alkalosis. ECG: normal.
Imaging	CXR (after patient stabilizes): **right pneumothorax compressing lung parenchyma and shifting of mediastinum toward left.** Flattened left hemidiaphragm.
Gross Pathology	Pleural space is filled with air and lung is atelectatic (to demonstrate pneumothorax at autopsy, the chest cavity is opened under water, letting air bubbles escape).
Micro Pathology	Section of lung shows collapsed alveolar spaces.
Treatment	Immediate life-saving treatment consists of inserting a wide-bore IV cannula on the affected side to decompress the pleural cavity if a chest drain is not immediately available; the wide-bore needle can then be replaced by a chest drain connected to an underwater seal.
Discussion	In tension pneumothorax, air enters the pleural space during inspiration and is prevented from escaping during expiration (because an airway or tissue flap acts as a one-way valve); there is a progressive increase in pleural air, which is under pressure (i.e., tension). Tension pneumothorax occurs in only 1% to 2% of cases of idiopathic spontaneous pneumothorax; it is a more common manifestation of the barotrauma that may occur during positive pressure mechanical ventilation. Risk factors for spontaneous pneumothorax include COPD, cystic fibrosis, asthma, and tuberculosis.

ID/CC	A **34-year-old** white obese **female** complains of **shortness of breath**, dizziness, and near-fainting spells.
HPI	She has been taking **prescription medication** for approximately 6 months in order to **lose weight**.
PE	Obesity; mild cyanosis; **large "a" wave** in jugular venous pressure; parasternal heave; **loud S2**; narrow splitting of S2; rales on both bases; hepatomegaly.
Labs	CBC: **polycythemia**. ECG: **right-axis deviation; right ventricle and right atrial hypertrophy**. ABGs: hypoxemia.
Imaging	CXR: enlarged right ventricle; enlarged main pulmonary artery with peripheral pruning.
Gross Pathology	Enlarged right ventricle with myocardial fiber hypertrophy; atherosclerosis of pulmonary artery; narrowing of arterioles.
Micro Pathology	Atheromas in main elastic arteries. Thickening of the media and intima in medium size muscular arteries, causing near-obliteration of the lumen.
Treatment	Calcium channel blockers; prostacyclin; inhaled nitric oxide; phlebotomy; heart-lung transplantation can be considered.
Discussion	Primary pulmonary hypertension is a pathologic increase in pulmonary artery pressure; if long-standing, it causes fatal right heart failure. It may be primary (idiopathic) or secondary to intrinsic pulmonary disease.
Atlas Link	ⓊⒸⓋⓘ PG-P2-090

ID/CC	A 60-year-old female who had undergone right **total hip replacement** presents on the sixth postoperative day with central **chest pain** and **acute-onset dyspnea**.
HPI	She has been **immobile** since the surgery.
PE	VS: low-grade fever; tachycardia; **tachypnea; hypotension**. PE: central cyanosis; **elevated JVP; right ventricular gallop rhythm with widely split S2**.
Labs	ABGs: **hypoxia and hypercapnia** (type 2 respiratory failure). ECG: **S1Q3T3** pattern and sinus **tachycardia**.
Imaging	US, Doppler: **clot in right common femoral vein**. CXR: right lower lobe atelectasis. V/Q: three areas of ventilation-perfusion mismatch in right lung. Angio, pulmonary: confirmatory; not required if V/Q scan is high probability.
Gross Pathology	Large thrombus seen in pulmonary artery.
Micro Pathology	Large occlusive thrombus seen in pulmonary artery with variable degree of recanalization.
Treatment	Supportive; thrombolytic therapy; consider embolectomy; heparin, Coumadin, and low-molecular-weight heparin (enoxaparin) instituted for prophylaxis (monitor INR).
Discussion	Pulmonary emboli most commonly originate from proximal deep venous thrombosis. Pulmonary angiography is the gold standard in the diagnosis of pulmonary embolism, but obtain a V/Q scan initially if clinically suspected. **Virchow's triad** outlines the risk factors for thrombus formation and includes blood stasis (e.g., immobilization), endothelial damage (e.g., surgery), and hypercoagulable states (e.g., malignancy, pregnancy, severe burns). Large emboli may cause cardiovascular collapse and sudden death.
Atlas Links	UCV1 PG-P2-091, PM-P2-091

ID/CC	A **28-year-old black female** complains of **fever, dyspnea, arthralgia, and erythematous, tender nodules** on both legs.
HPI	She has no history of foreign travel or contact with a tubercular patient.
PE	VS: fever. PE: tender, **erythematous nodules over extensor aspects of both legs** (ERYTHEMA NODOSUM); arthralgias of both knees; splenomegaly.
Labs	CBC: **lymphopenia; eosinophilia**. Lytes: **elevated serum calcium; hypercalciuria. ACE levels elevated**; blood cultures negative; **Mantoux test negative**; fungal serology negative. PFTs: **evidence of restrictive changes**. Transbronchial lung biopsy ordered.
Imaging	CXR: **bilateral hilar lymphadenopathy** and right paratracheal adenopathy; **interstitial infiltrates**; no pleural effusion.
Gross Pathology	Firm nodules only a few millimeters in size in affected organs; can become confluent and give rise to larger nodules.
Micro Pathology	Lymph node biopsy reveals **noncaseating granulomas** with fibrotic acellular core surrounded by lymphocytes, epithelioid cells, and Langerhan's giant cells.
Treatment	**Corticosteroids**.
Discussion	In the United States, the incidence of sarcoidosis is highest in black women, with onset between 20 and 40 years of age. The disease may be asymptomatic; however, symptoms may be constitutional and may involve many different organ systems, including the lungs, lymph nodes, skin, eye, upper respiratory tract, reticuloendothelial system, liver, kidneys, nervous system, and heart. Approximately 60% to 70% of sarcoidosis patients recover with few or no residual symptoms.
Atlas Link	UCVI PM-P2-092

ID/CC	A 56-year-old male presents with progressively increasing **dyspnea** and **dry cough** of several years' duration.
HPI	He is a nonsmoker, but his occupational history includes **mining and quarrying**.
PE	No clubbing, cyanosis, or lymphadenopathy; **reduced chest expansion** on inspiration; **dry inspiratory crackles** auscultated in upper lobes of both lungs.
Labs	PFTs: combined **obstructive and restrictive pattern** of functional impairment. Bronchoscopically-guided lung biopsy establishes diagnosis; negative Mantoux test; sputum cytology and staining for acid-fast bacilli negative.
Imaging	CXR, PA: rounded small opacities in upper lobes with retraction and **hilar lymphadenopathy; "eggshell" calcification of lymph nodes**.
Gross Pathology	Dense, small collagenous nodules in the upper lungs in the early stages; spread and become more diffuse as disease progresses.
Micro Pathology	Hyalinized whorls of collagen with little or no inflammation; polarized light demonstrates silica particles within nodules.
Treatment	Supportive; avoidance of further exposure.
Discussion	There is an **increased incidence of tuberculosis** in silicosis patients. Silicosis leads to restrictive lung disease that varies in severity from mild to disabling.
Atlas Link	UCVI PG-P2-093

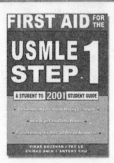
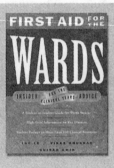
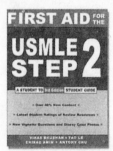
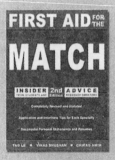